HANDBOOK

OF

OPHTHALMIC
INSTRUMENTS

HANDBOOK

OF

OPHTHALMIC
INSTRUMENTS

Dr. Anita Panda

MD, FAMS, FICO, FICS, MRCOphth.

Former Professor & HOD, Cornea and Ocular Surface Disorders,
Dr. RP Centre for Ophthalmic Sciences, AIIMS, New Delhi

Past President, All India Ophthalmological Society

Former Professor, Deptt. of Ophthalmology, Sharda University, Greater Noida, UP

Dr. Abhiyan Kumar

DOMS, FMRF (Sankara Nethralaya, Chennai)

Director, Dr. Pattnaik's Laser Eye Institute, New Delhi

Dr. Rasheena Bansal

DNB, MNAMS, FICO

Senior Consultant, Paediatric Ophthalmology,
Dr. Pattnaik's Laser Eye Institute, New Delhi

Foreword by

Joel Sugar, MD

Professor of Ophthalmology, Vice Chair, Clinical Operations,
Illinois Eye and Infirmary, Chicago, USA

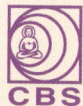

CBS Publishers & Distributors Pvt. Ltd.

New Delhi • Bengaluru • Chennai • Kochi • Kolkata • Mumbai
Hyderabad • Nagpur • Patna • Pune • Vijayawada

ISBN: 978-93-86478-57-3

First Edition: 2017

Published by **Satish Kumar Jain** and produced by **Varun Jain** for **CBS Publishers & Distributors Pvt. Ltd.,**
4819/XI Prahlad Street, 24 Ansari Road, Daryaganj, New Delhi - 110002
delhi@cbspd.com, cbspubs@airtelmail.in • www.cbspd.com
Ph.: 23289259, 23266861, 23266867 • Fax: 011-23243014

Corporate Office: 204 FIE, Industrial Area, Patparganj, Delhi - 110 092
Ph: 49344934 • Fax: 011-49344935
E-mail: publishing@cbspd.com • publicity@cbspd.com

Branches:
• *Bengaluru:* 2975, 17th Cross, K.R. Road, Bansankari 2nd Stage, Bengaluru - 70 • Ph: +91-80-26771678/79 • Fax: +91-80-26771680
E-mail: cbsbng@gmail.com, bangalore@cbspd.com
• *Chennai:* No. 7, Subbaraya Street, Shenoy Nagar, Chennai - 600030
Ph: +91-44-26681266, 26680620 • Fax: +91-44-42032115
E-mail: chennai@cbspd.com
• *Kochi:* Ashana House, 39/1904, A.M. Thomas Road, Valanjambalam, Ernakulum, Kochi • Ph: +91-484-4059061-65
Fax: +91-484-4059065 • E-mail: cochin@cbspd.com
• *Kolkata:* 6-B, Ground Floor, Rameshwar Shaw Road, Kolkata - 700014
Ph: +91-33-22891126/7/8 • E-mail: kolkata@cbspd.com
• *Mumbai:* 83-C, Dr. E. Moses Road, Worli, Mumbai - 400018
Ph: +91-9833017933, 022-24902340/41 • E-mail: mumbai@cbspd.com

Representatives:
• Hyderabad: 0-9885175004   • Nagpur: 0-9021734563
• Patna: 0-9334159340   • Pune: 0-9623451994
• Vijayawada: 0-9000660880

Printed at:
India Binding House, Noida (U.P.), India

*Dedicated to
my
beloved students*

FOREWORD

One of the basic essentials of all technologic enterprises, surgery included, is the need to "know your tools". Dr. Panda and her co-authors of this book take on the important challenge of reviewing the wide array of tools (instruments) that we, as ophthalmic surgeons, need to be, or become, familiar with. The surgeon, in turn, must select from these multiple options the tools that best meet her or his needs. Factors that must be considered include function, versatility, durability, availability, and cost among others. The number of variables for each type of instrument can at times appear overwhelming and, for example, in forceps, can include handle type – round, flat; locking, spring-held; tip type – straight, angled; tooth design – "rat toothed", serrated, flat; tooth number – 2:1, 3:2; overall size; metallic composition; and many others to incompletely name a few. Each surgeon must become familiar with the available instruments, their functional capabilities and their subtleties and then develop ideally the smallest set of tools that meets his/her needs for each type of procedure. Failure to become aware of the spectrum of instruments limits the potential to provide optimal patient care.

Dr. Panda, an exceptionally experienced ophthalmic surgeon and teacher, is well equipped to carry out this difficult task and succeeds in this work in making our choices easier and better. Her product is one to be proud of. Not only will this assist students, trainees, and practitioners presently in the field, but can serve as a basis for the development of even better instruments for our practice in the future.

Dr. Joel Sugar MD
Professor of Ophthalmology,
Vice Chair, Clinical Operations,
Illinois Eye and Ear Infirmary, Chicago

PREFACE

The present book on "Ophthalmic Instruments" is designed for medical students; ophthalmic technique students; postgraduate students in ophthalmology, who are at their learning stage and also budding Ophthalmic Practitioners to select the instruments for their practice to form the basic ground-work for subsequent practice.

Over the years, it has been learnt that although proper instruments and equipments go a long way for the clinical examination, the concise book is lacking. This book is the experience of the authors over years in the field of ophthalmology.

At the medical colleges, this was the constant request from each batch of MBBS students to have a separate instrument book. Later, when I was President of All India Ophthalmological Society, I was travelling a lot to establish the standard postgraduate teaching all over the country. This request had also arose from PG and DNB students to make an exclusive ophthalmic instruments book available. This book is the outcome.

Section I deals with the general ophthalmic instruments, and Section II highlights the set of instruments required for specific surgeries.

It is assumed that the learners will have a better understanding on the ophthalmic instruments as a whole and will apply the same in their practice.

The text is lucid and concise, yet, comprehensive. Finally, this book will be useful "as a guide manual" to the medical students, ophthalmic residents in training, budding ophthalmologists to establish their operation theatre and also ophthalmic practitioners. Besides, it will also serve as a guide manual for governmental and non-governmental organizations to provide aid for the unequipped hospitals, public health centres and alike.

Suggestions for using this book

This book is structured in such a way so that each instrument is kept in separate group and again in a selective way to be dealt with the different structures of ophthalmic surgery.

Dr. Anita Panda

ACKNOWLEDGEMENTS

I am very grateful to the Almighty for enabling me to complete this book.

This book would not have been possible without the help and encouragement of numerous individuals from home and abroad.

First and foremost, my thanks must go to my patients, past and present, who were the source for increasing my experience and knowledge in the field of ophthalmology. I humbly place on record my concern for those on whose eyes I have performed various ophthalmic surgeries which made me wise to select proper instruments to be used for a particular ocular tissue during specific surgery.

My sincere gratitude to Dr. L.P. Agarwal, the former Chief of Dr. R.P. Center and former Director of AIIMS for introducing me to ophthalmology.

I appreciate the encouragement of Dr. Kulamani Mishra, my teacher, who encouraged me to undertake ophthalmology.

I express my thanks to Appasamy Associates for providing me many photographs.

I am especially appreciative and greatly indebted to Dr. Abhiyan Kumar, co-author of the book, for his active help in getting the photographs and critical comments on the need of students' requirements in present era which have made the book more lively.

I also appreciate the work of Dr. Rasheena, a co-author, for her editing and untiring efforts to bring together the myriad of details necessary for publishing the book.

Individually, I thank the little Adu who increased my concentration of finishing the long-waiting book.

And finally, I am grateful to Dr Joel Sugar for his kind words.

Dr. Anita Panda

CONTENTS

Section 1

GENERAL
OPHTHALMIC
INSTRUMENTS

OPHTHALMIC INSTRUMENTS

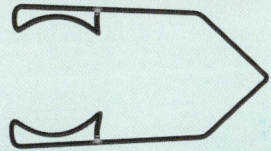

"Speculum" is the instrument to keep the lids wide apart to provide better exposure of the eye.

Types

1. Universal eye speculum
   • Heavy instrument and cannot keep eyelashes out of the operating field.
2. Guarded eye speculum (left and right)
   • Heavy instrument but can keep eyelashes out of the operating field with its "guard" and hence left or right ones are required.
3. Wire speculum
   • Light wire instrument.

Uses

Eye speculums are used to keep the lids apart during:

1. Any intraocular operation such as cataract surgery and glaucoma surgery and so on.
2. Any extraocular surgery, e.g., squint surgery, pterygium surgery and so on.
3. Enucleation and evisceration operation.
4. Removal of conjunctival and corneal foreign bodies.
5. Cauterization of corneal ulcer.
6. Examination of the eye in a patient with blepharospasm and a child's eye.

Types of Speculum

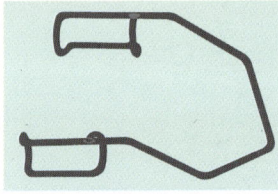

Barraquer wire speculum

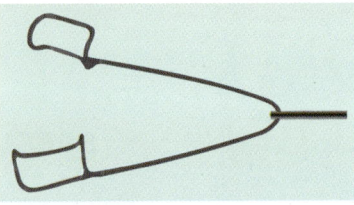

Pannu-Barraquer aspirating speculum

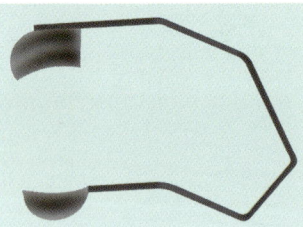

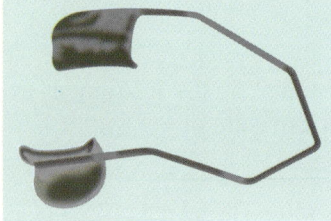

Barraquer wire speculum with solid blades

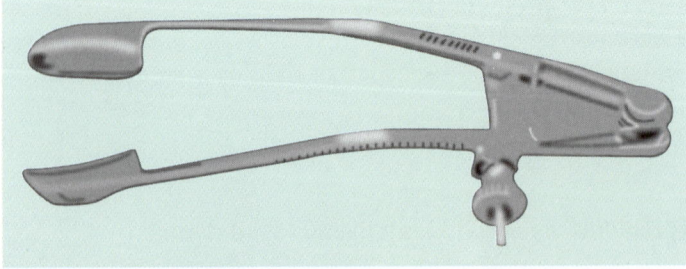

Lancaster speculum with solid blades

RETRACTORS

To pull and hold overlying tissue out of the operating field or especially for noncooperative patients and to see the fornices.

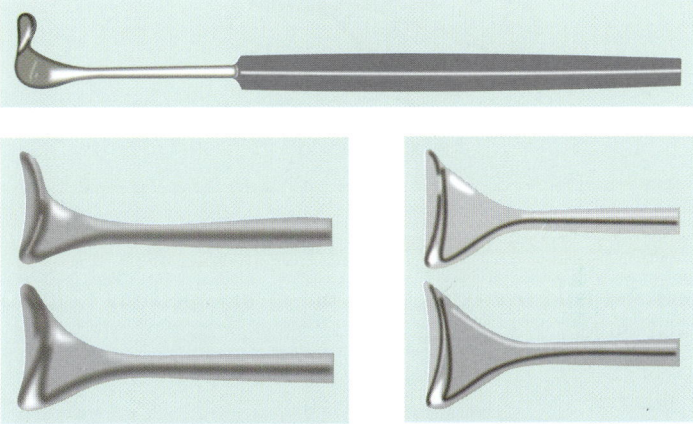

Desmarres lid retractors with solid blades

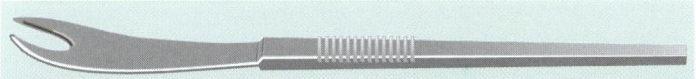

Schepens forked orbital retractor

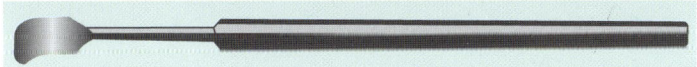

Helveston tissue retractor with thin curved blades

Self-Retaining Lacrimal Wound (Muller's) Retractor

- It is made up of two limbs with three curved pins on each for engaging the edges of the skin incision.
- The limbs are kept in a retracted position with the help of a fixing screw.

Uses

- It is used to retract the skin during surgery on the lacrimal sac (e.g., DCT or DCR).

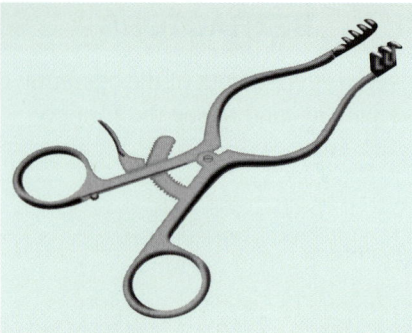

Cat's Paw Retractor

To pull and hold overlying tissue out of the operating field during lacrimal surgery.

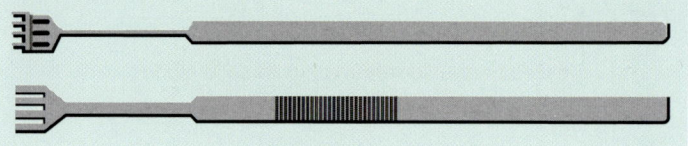

CLAMPS

Lid Clamp or Entropion Clamp

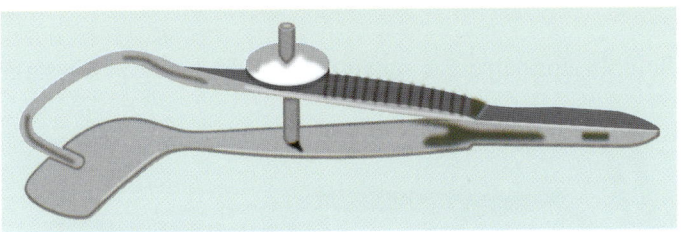

Snellen's entropion clamp, left upper, right lower

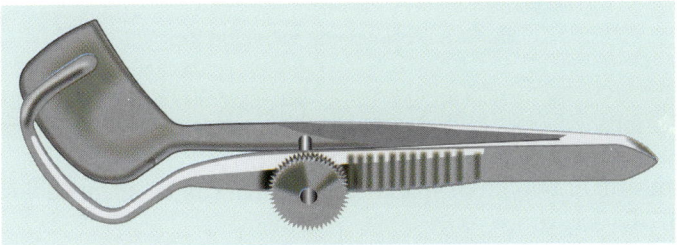

Snellen's entropion clamp, right upper, left lower

Types

- Right and left varieties exist.
- Large clamp with two limbs.
- Self-retaining with big discoid ends used to hold and prevent an entropion from bleeding during its surgery.

Advantage over lid spatula

- It is a self-retaining instrument and does not need an assistant to hold.

Disadvantages

1. Operative field is less.
2. Pressure necrosis can occur if fitted tightly (rare).

Uses

- It is used in lid surgery, e.g., entropion and ectropion corrections.
- It protects the eyeball, supports the lid tissue and provides haemostasis during surgery.

Ptosis Clamp

- It is like forceps with J-shaped ends having internal serrations.
- The clamp has a locking mechanism.

Uses

- To hold levator palpebrae superioris muscle during ptosis surgery.

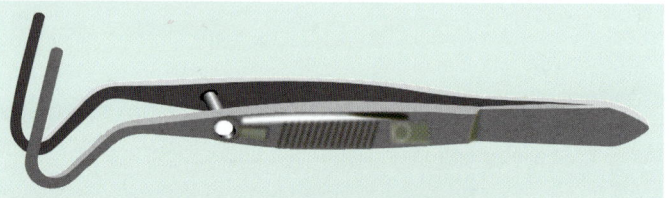

Berke's ptosis clamp with side lock

Chalazion Clamp

- It consists of two limbs like forceps, which can be clamped with the help of a screw.
- The tip of one limb is flattened in the form of round disc while the tip of the other arm has a small circular ring.
- The flat disc is applied on the skin side and ring on the conjunctival side of the chalazion when approached from conjunctival side and vice versa.

Uses

- To fix the chalazion and achieve haemostasis during incision and curettage.

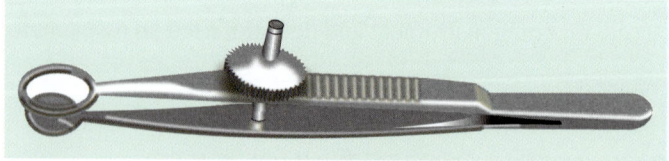

Ayer chalazion clamp

Lid Guard

Flat large instrument that has a groove and is placed between the lid and globe of the eye to provide a solid support for eyelid surgery.

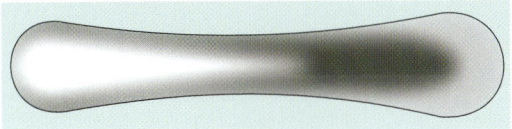

Jaeger lid plate

Fixation Rings

These are round rings used for fixing the globe for various surgeries.

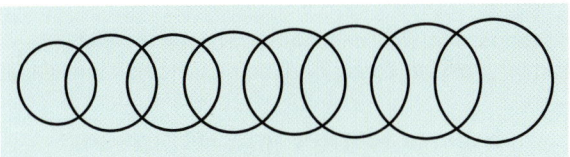

Fleiringa scleral fixation rings

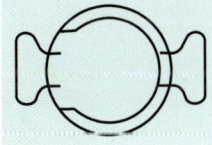

Goldmann scleral fixation rings

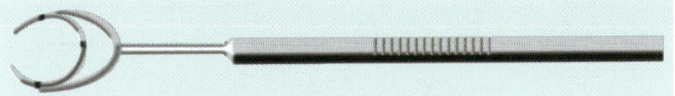

Shepard fixation ring for clear corneal incision

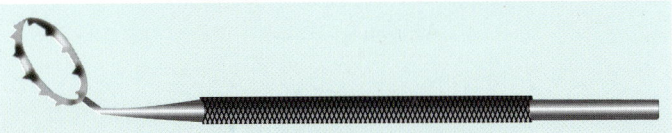

Thompton globe fixation ring

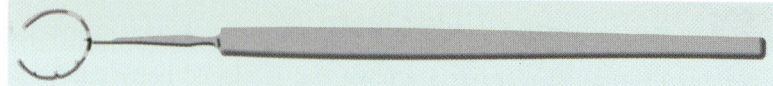

Thompton globe fixation ring, open

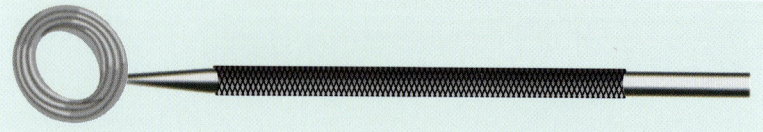

Appasamy fixation ring with concentric grooves for stabilising globe during PRK and LASIK surgery

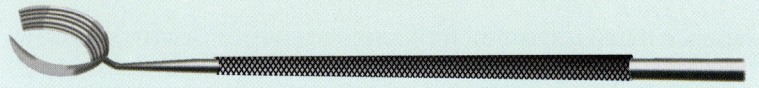

Appasamy fixation ring with concentric grooves for stabilising globe and providing counter-pressure during clear corneal incision and IOL insertion

Scleral Marker and Depressor

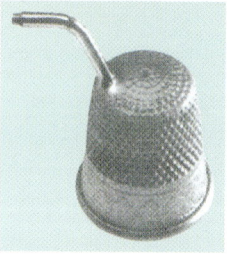

Gass scleral marker

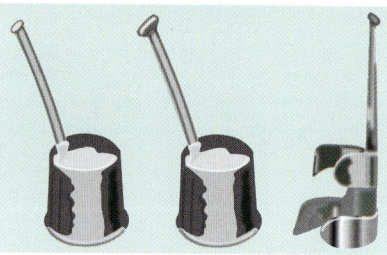

Schepens scleral depressor

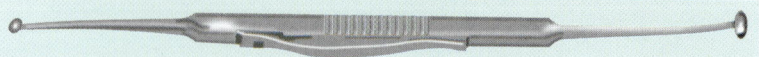

Shocket scleral depresser double end with pocket clip

CAUTERY

Thermocautery

- To cauterise the bleeding vessels.

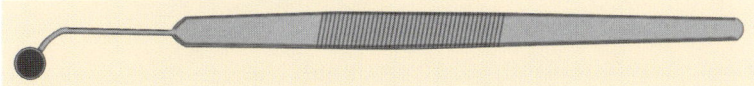

Electric Cautery (Bipolar)

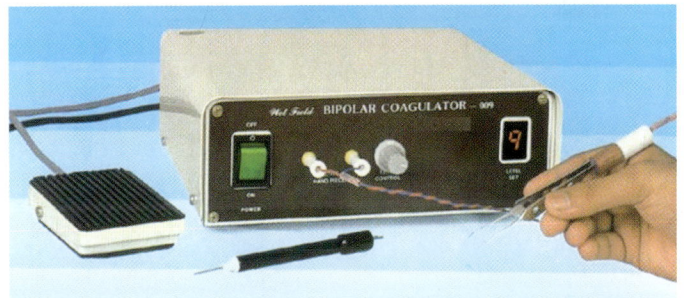

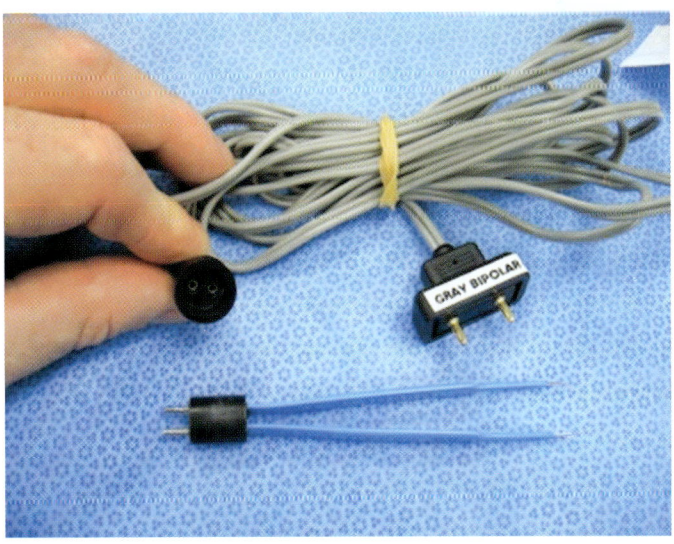

Bipolar Cautery

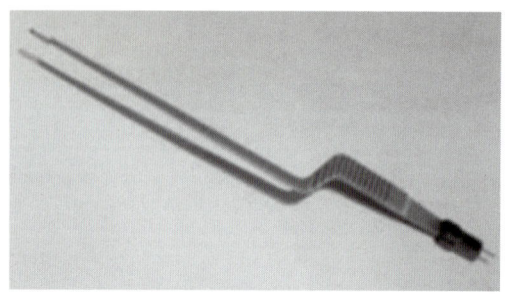

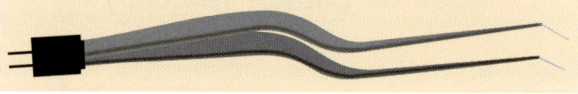

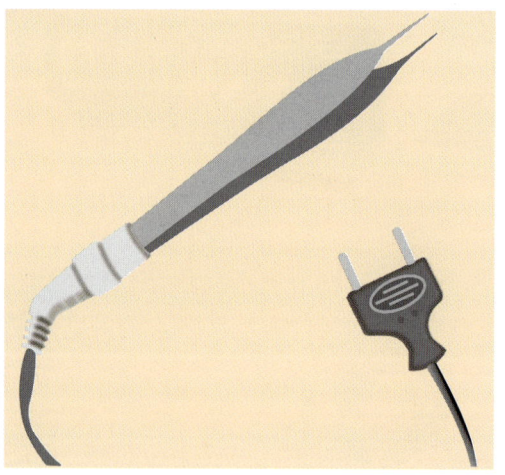

FORCEPS

To hold tissues and linens commonly known as towel clip.

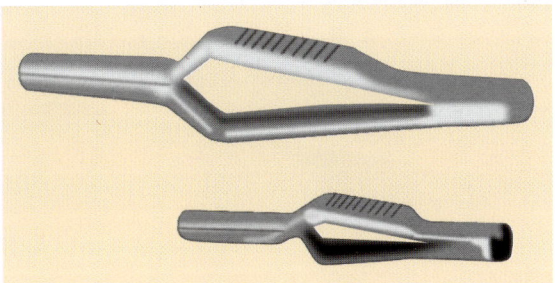

Artery Forceps

- Medium-sized, with a serrated tip and a catch.
- Used to hold bleeding vessels and compress them to make them stop bleeding and also to hold or crush structures.

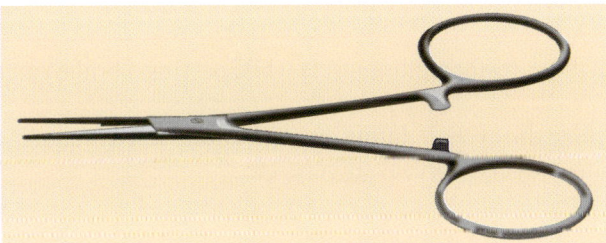

Hartman mosquito forceps

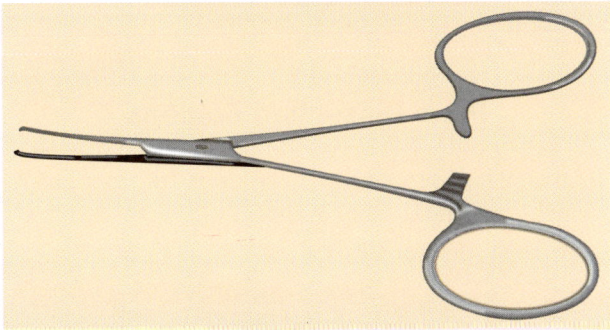

Allis tissue forceps

Fixation Forceps

Has a few teeth at the tip for holding structures and restricting their movement or to hold small swabs.

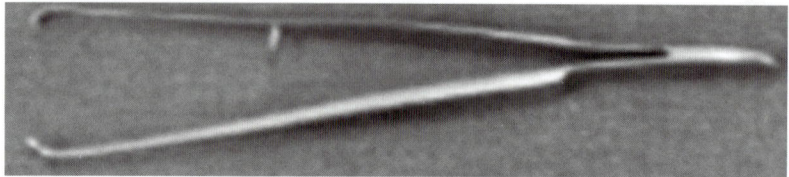

Superior Rectus Holding Forceps

S-shaped double curve near the tip.

Toothed Forceps

- It is specially curved forceps (to fit into the orbit of the eyeball) for catching hold of the muscle bellies of the superior rectus muscle.

Uses

- To hold the superior rectus muscle while passing a bridle suture under it.
- To stabilize the eyeball during any operation such as cataract surgery, glaucoma surgery, corneal surgery, etc.

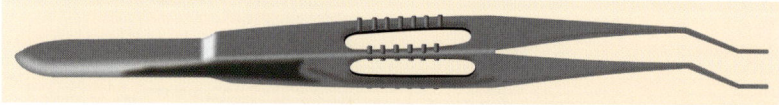

Plain Dissecting Forceps

Blunt untoothed with a serrated tip for holding structures and restricting their movement or to hold small swabs.

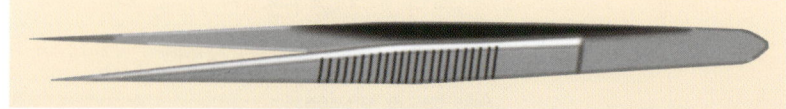

Corneal Forceps

Corneoscleral forceps

Uses

- These are used to hold the cornea or scleral edge (of incision) for suturing during cataract, glaucoma, repair of corneal and/or scleral tears and keratoplasty operations.

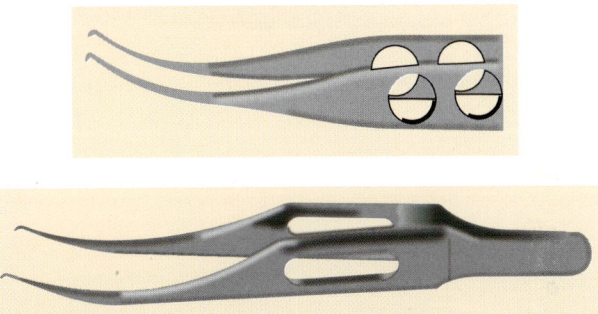

Colibri Forceps

Fine-toothed forceps for holding flaps of cornea or sclera and rarely the iris.

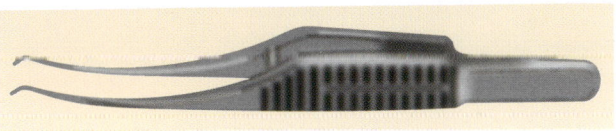

Barraquer Colibri forceps

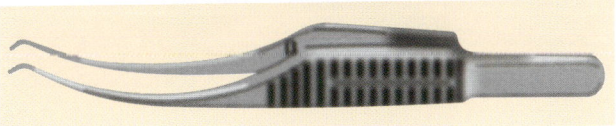

Gill Colibri forceps

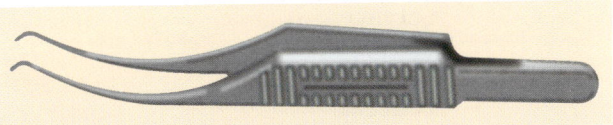

Harms Colibri forceps

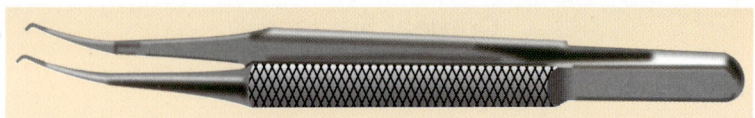

Birk Colibri forceps

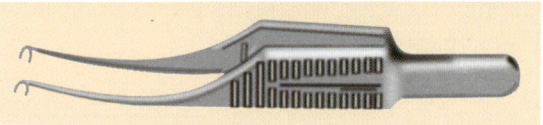

Polack double corneal forceps specially designed to hold the tissue during keratoplasty

Pierse Forceps

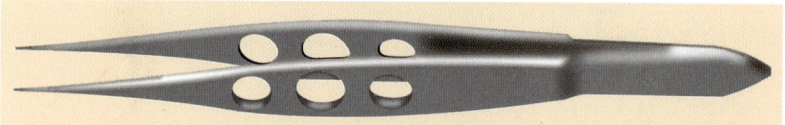

Pierse corneal forceps

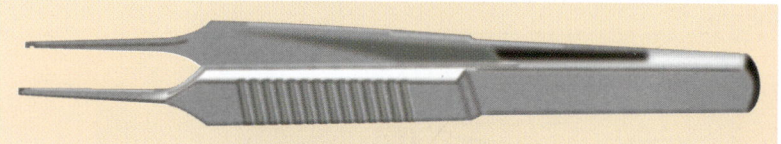

Pierse type microforceps, straight

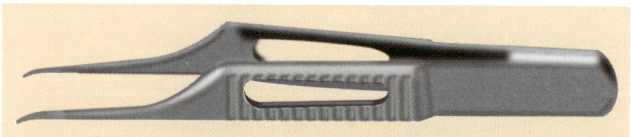

Pierse type microforceps, curved

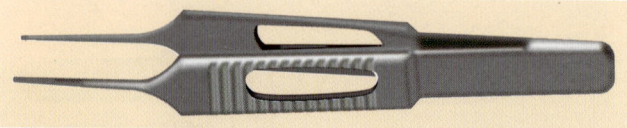

Pierse type microforceps, straight skeleton, fine

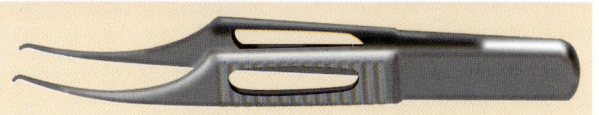

Pierse type microforceps beaked, fine colibri

Lim's Forceps

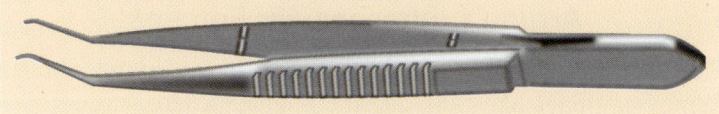

Lim's corneoscleral forceps with tying platform

Iris Forceps

- Fine-tipped (straight or otherwise) with small teeth.
- To hold the iris tissue during procedures.

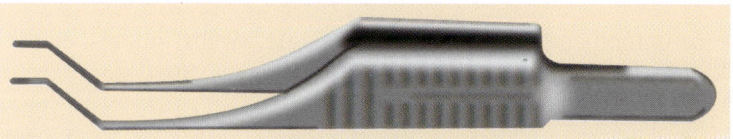

Botvin iris forceps

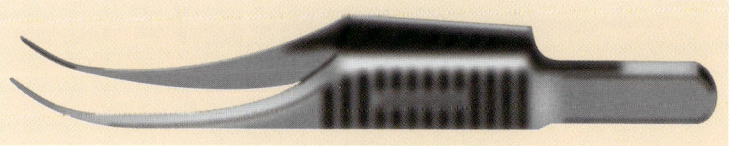

Gill's iris forceps, curved

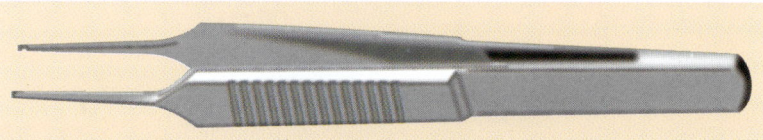

Swiss model iris forceps, curved, delicate

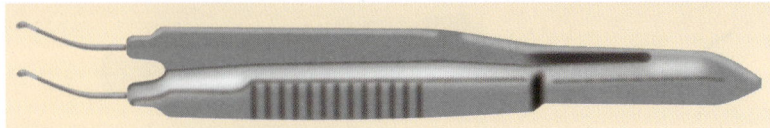

Hess iris forceps, standard model

Intracapsular Forceps

Arruga's Intracapsular Forceps

- Fine untoothed forceps for holding tissue, swabs, sutures, etc.
- Removing things like clots, capsule fragments, lens, etc.
- Used in cataract surgery.

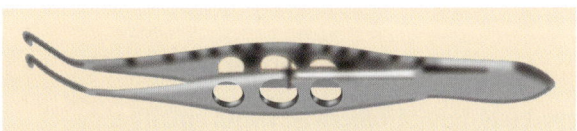

Elschnig's Intracapsular Forceps

- Fine untoothed forceps for holding tissue, swabs, sutures, etc.
- Removing things like clots, capsule fragments, lens, etc.
- Used in cataract surgery.

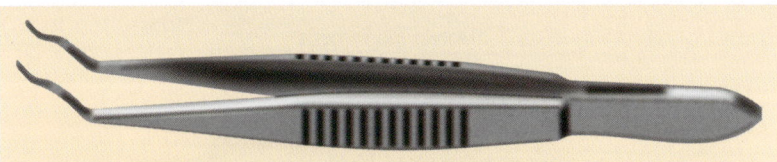

Capsulorhexis Forceps

Fine sharp-tipped untoothed forceps for doing a continuous curvilinear incision and removal of the anterior capsule of the lens ("Continuous Curvilinear Capsulorhexis – CCC") prior to cataract surgery.

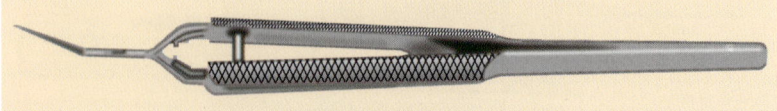

Akahoshi capsulorhexis forceps

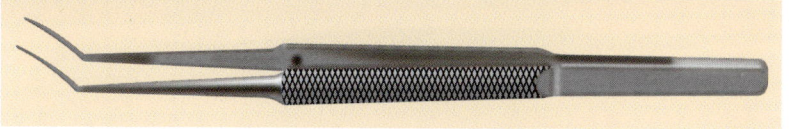

Utrata capsulorhexis forceps

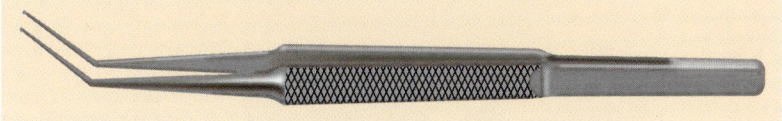

Pierce capsulorhexis forceps

IOL Holding Forceps

It is a spring action forceps with short, blunt and curved blades having smooth edges and tips with plateform (no teeth or serrations).

Uses

To hold optic of non-foldable PMMA IOL during implantation.

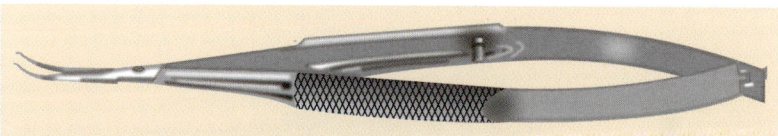

Kraff lens holding forceps

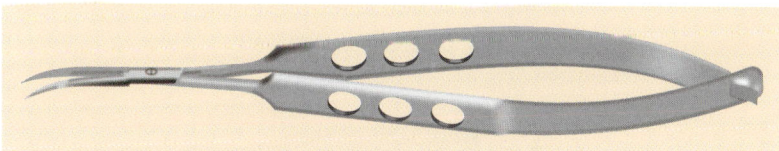

Kratz lens holding forceps

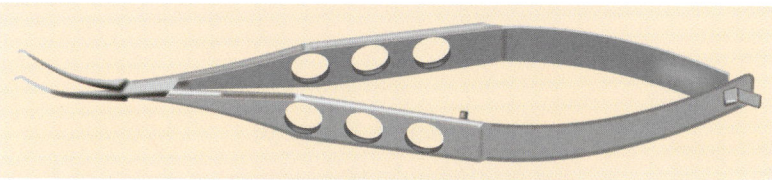

Clayman lens holding forceps

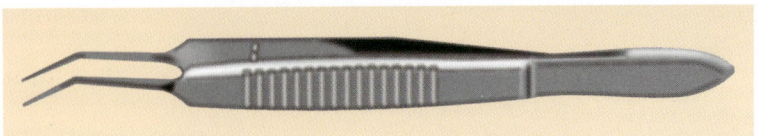

Dodick lens holding forceps, smooth jaw

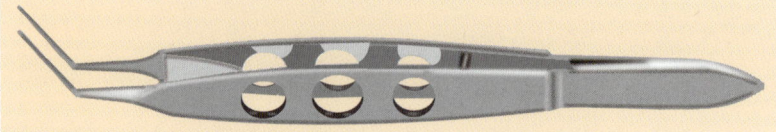

Kellan endocapsular lens holding forceps

Vitreous Forceps

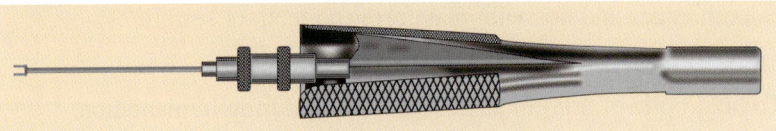

Vitreous forceps, smooth jaws

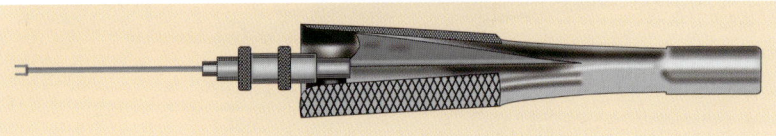

Vitreous forceps, serrated jaws

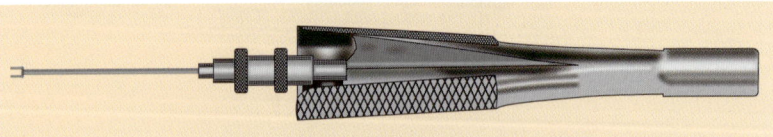

Vitreous forceps, smooth jaws – 1 in 2 tooth

McPherson Forceps

These are fine sharp-tipped untoothed forceps with an angulation (bent limbs).

Uses

1. To hold the superior haptic of IOL during its placement.
2. To tear off the anterior capsular flap in ECCE.
3. Can be used for suture tying.

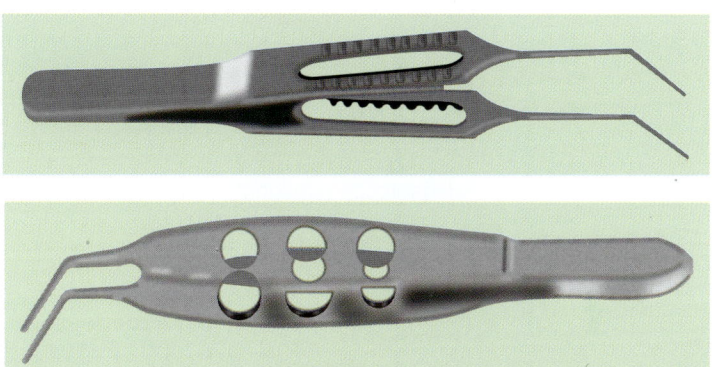

Tying Forceps

Fine-limbed untoothed forceps to hold fine sutures or hairs.

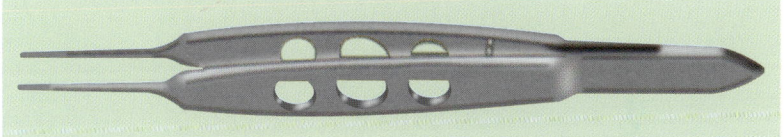

McPherson tying forceps, short handle

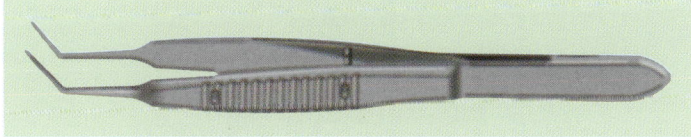

Kelman McPherson tying forceps, short handle

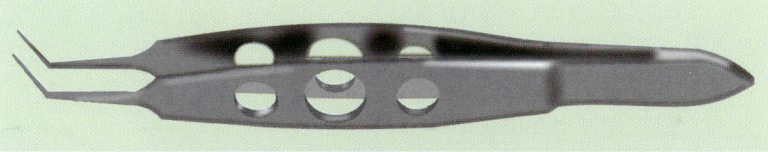

Kelman McPherson tying forceps, long handle

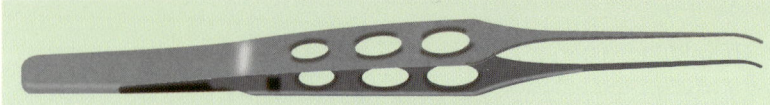

Tying forceps (curved)

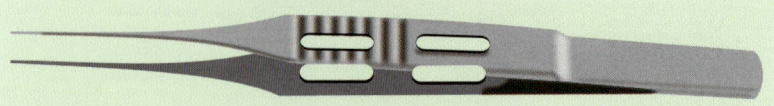

Tying forceps (straight)

Forceps for Muscle Surgery

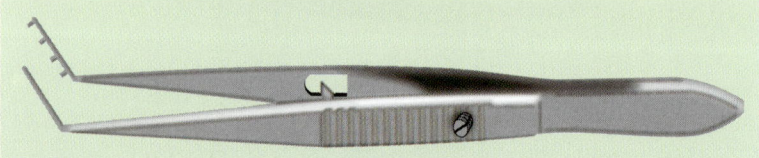

Prince advancement forceps, left

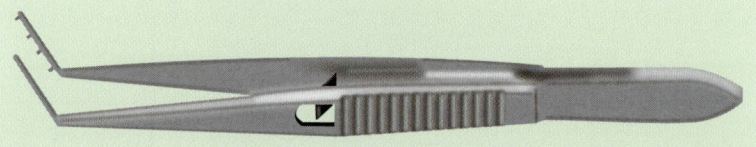

Prince advancement forceps, right

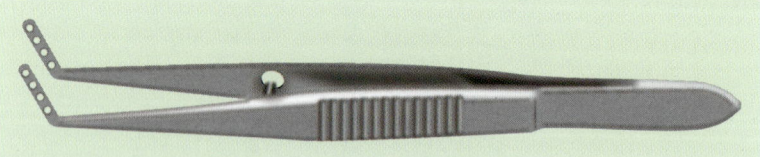

Jamesons muscle forceps with slide lock, 4 teeth, left

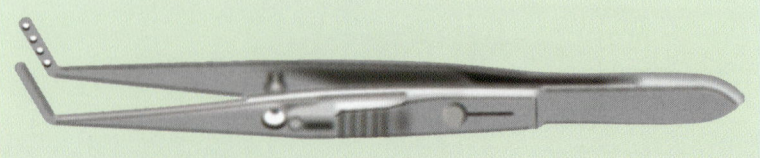

Jamesons muscle forceps with slide lock, 4 teeth, right

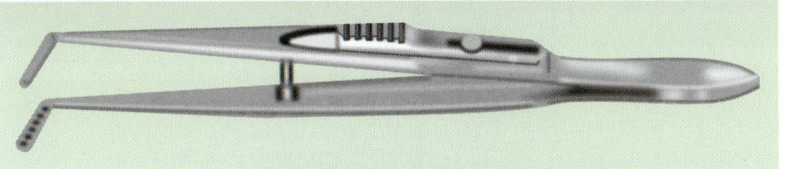

Jamesons muscle forceps with slide lock, 6 teeth, left

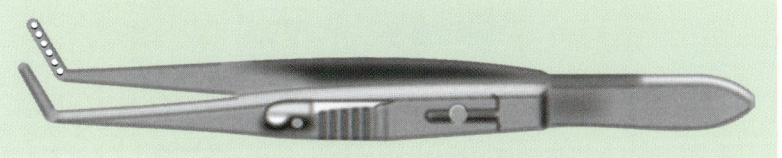

Jamesons muscle forceps with slide lock, 6 teeth, right

SCISSORS

Conjunctiva Scissors

Flat small curved scissors to cut the conjunctiva.

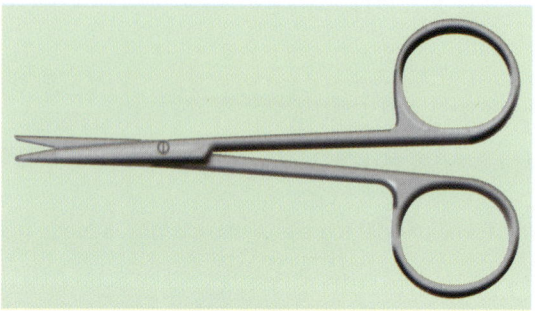

Corneal Scissors

Corneal scissors or section enlarging scissors.

Uses

• These are used to enlarge corneal or corneoscleral incision for conventional intracapsular and extracapsular cataract extraction (sparingly performed procedures now-a-days) cataract surgery.
• To enlarge corneal incision in keratoplasty operation.

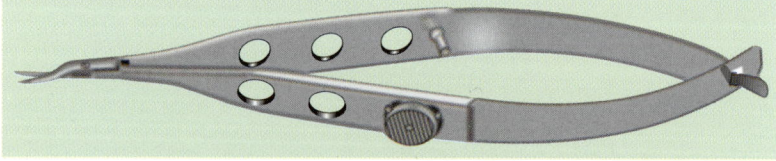

Troutman Katzan corneal transplant scissors, small blades

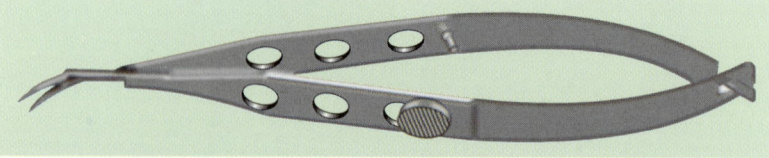

Troutman Katzan corneal transplant scissors, long blades

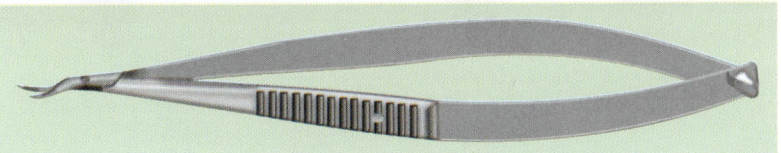

Castroviejo corneal scissors, small blade

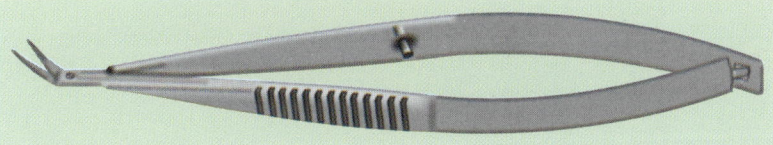

Castroviejo corneal scissors, small blade

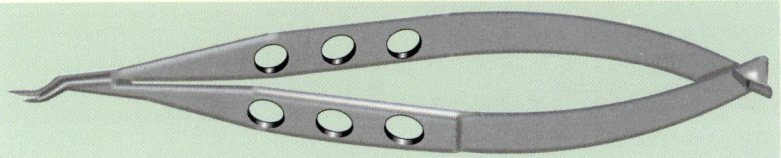

Castroviejo corneal scissors, medium blade

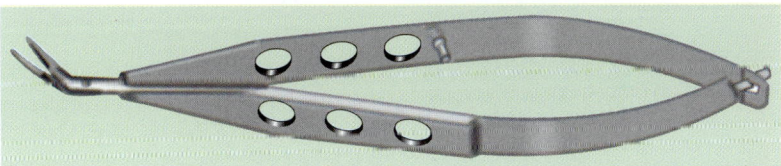

Castroviejo corneal scissors, medium blade

Corneal Spring Scissors

Medium spring-open scissors used to cut the external side of the cornea.

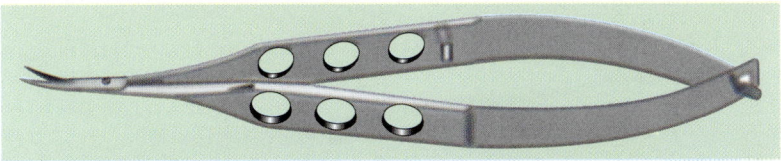

Castroviejo corneal scissors, curved blunt tip and small blades

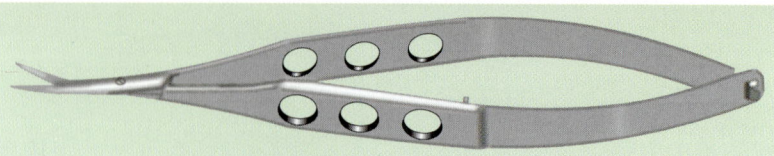

Castroviejo corneal scissors, curved blunt tip

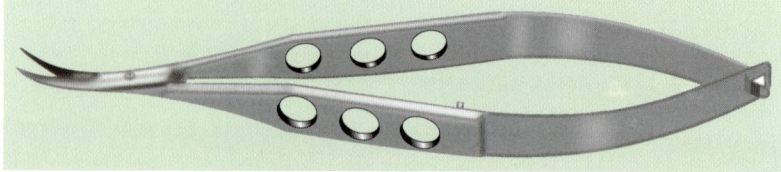

Castroviejo corneal transplant scissors

Vannas Scissors

- Small slender spring-open scissors for intraocular manoeuvres (iris and deeper and more delicate structures).
- Has two wings to operate it and one sharp and one blunt blade.

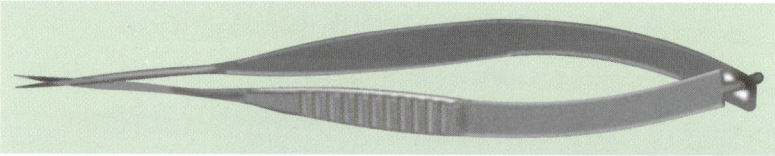

Vannas scissors, sharp pointed tip, straight

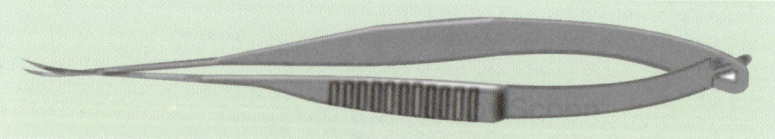

Vannas scissors, sharp pointed tip, curved

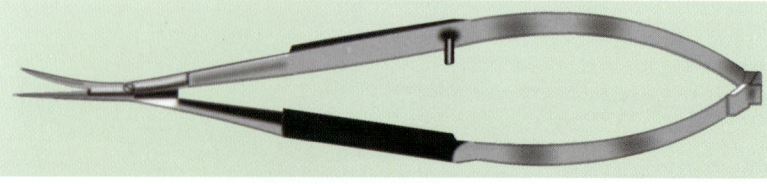

Vanna's scissors (straight)

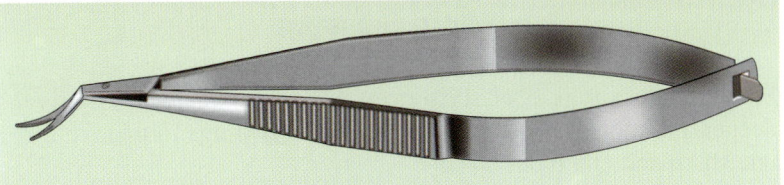

Vanna's scissors (angle)

Capsulotomy Scissors

To tear the anterior lens capsule during cataract surgery.

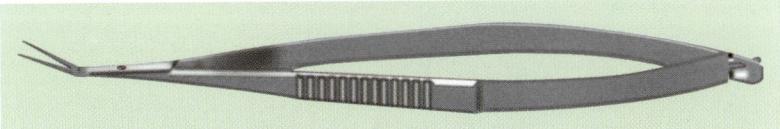

Stern-Gills capsulotomy scissors, thin, long and curve blade

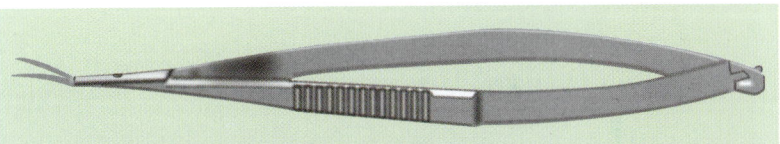

Hoffer Stern capsulotomy scissors, thin and curve blade

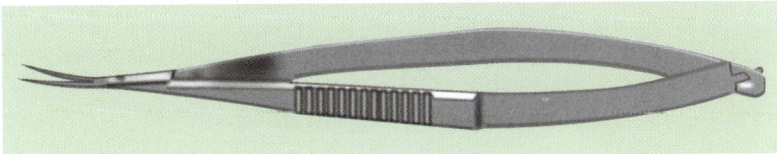

Urbe Stern capsulotomy scissors, extra thin and curve blade

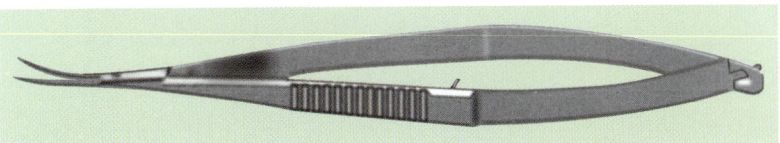

Koch endocapsular scissors, extra thin and curve blade

Micro Scissors

Small slender spring-open scissors for intraocular manoeuvres (iris and deeper and more delicate structures); has two wings to operate it and one sharp and one blunt blade.

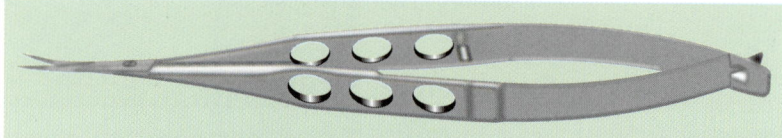

McPherson Westcott stitch scissors, sharp, pointed tip

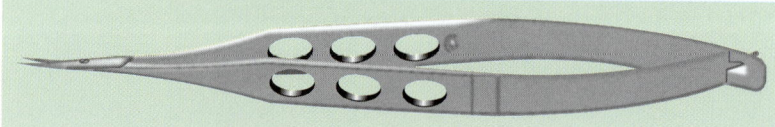

Jaffe stitch scissors, sharp pointed tip

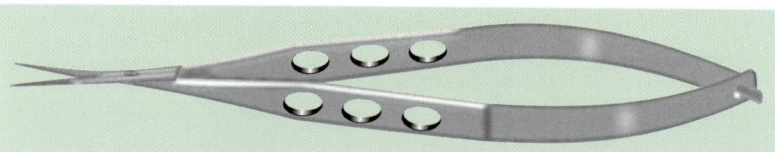

Fine stitch scissors, sharp pointed tip

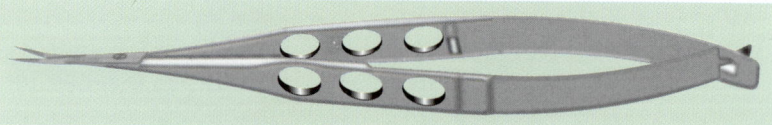

Westcott tenotomy scissors, curved, blunt tip

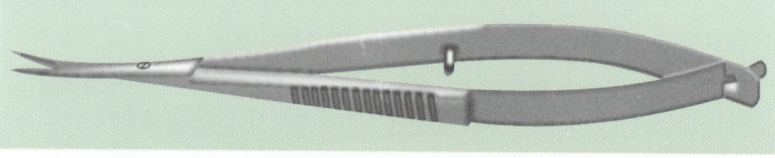

Westcott tenotomy scissors, curved, blunt tip, standard blade

de Wecker's Iris Scissors

They are fine scissors with small slender spring-open blades directed at right angles to the arms. The blades are kept apart, making V-shape, by spring action.

Uses

- It is used to perform iridectomy, iridotomy and to cut the prolapsed formed vitreous and pupillary membrane.

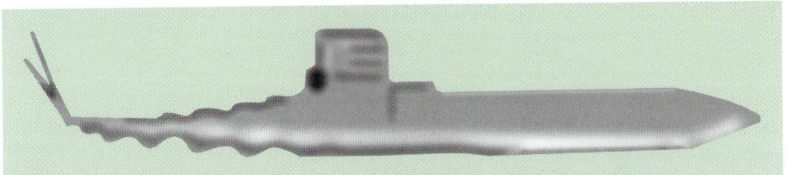

Scissors

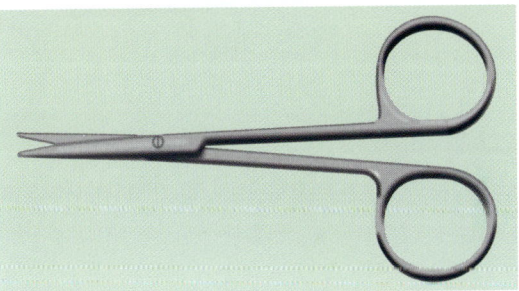

Knapp strabismus scissors, ring handle, straight

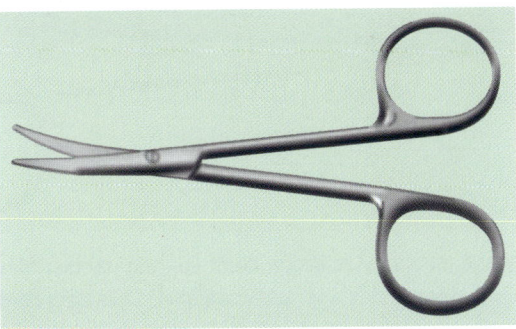

Knapp strabismus scissors, ring handle, curved

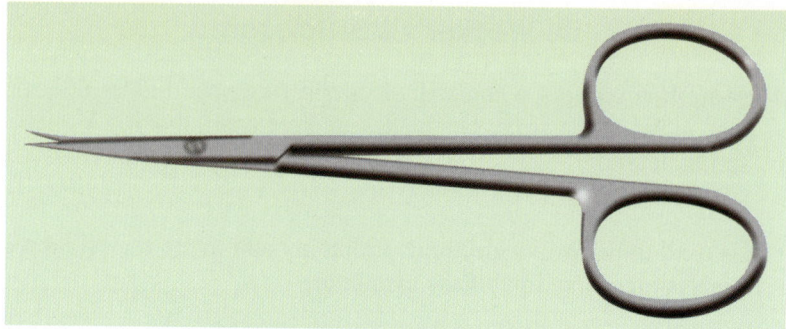

Stitch scissors, curved, ring handle

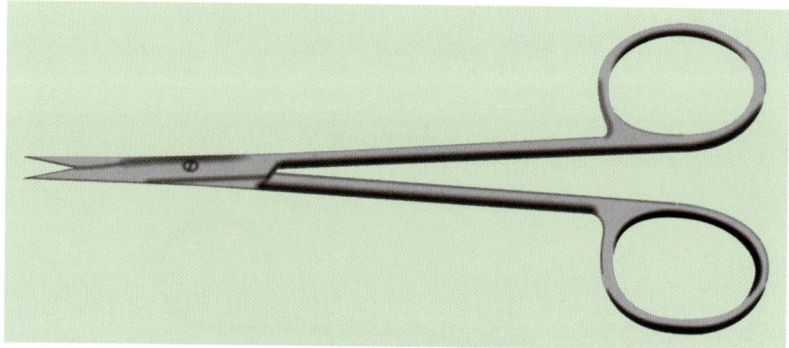

Stevens tenotomy scissors, blunt tip, ring handle, straight

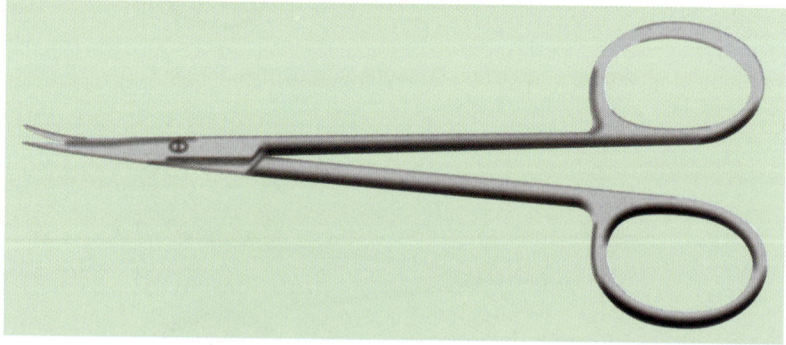

Stevens tenotomy scissors, blunt tip, ring handle, curved

Enucleation Scissors

Thick scissors used to cut the optic nerve during enucleation operation.

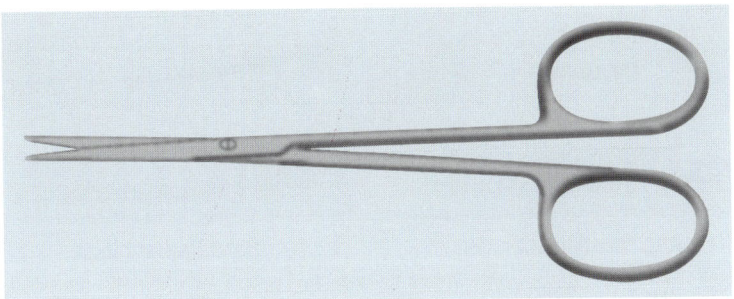

Enucleation scissors, ring handle, straight

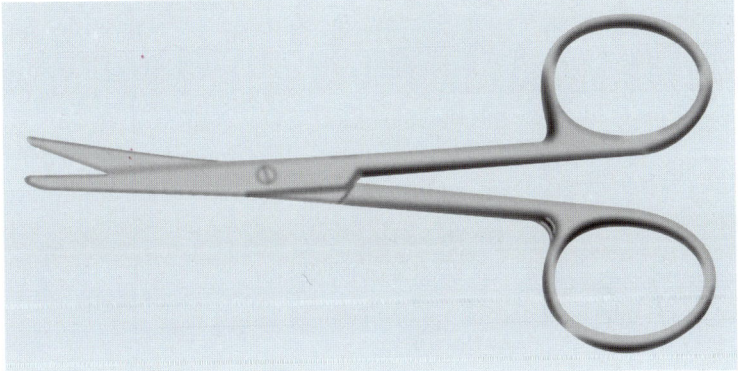

Enucleation scissors, ring handle, medium curved

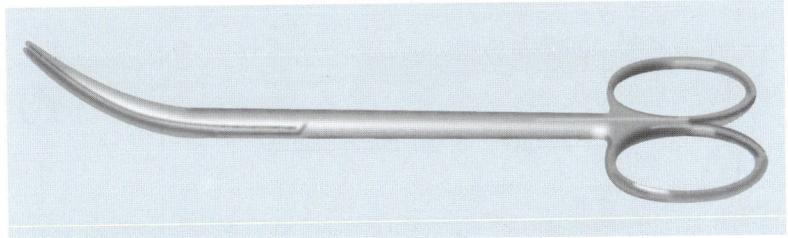

Enucleation scissors, ring handle, more curved

SURGICAL KNIVES, BLADES & BLADE BREAKERS

Blades

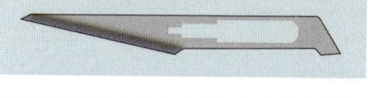
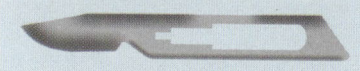

Surgical scalpel blade

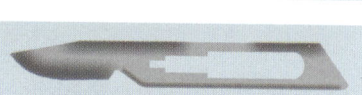

Bard Parker blade

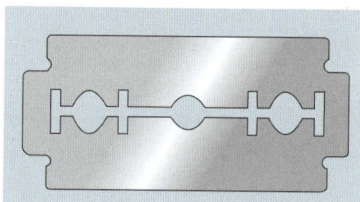

Carbon razor blade

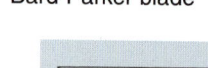
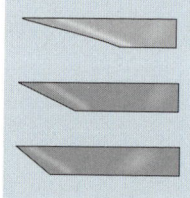

Pre-cut microblade fragment

Blade Breaker and Holder

• To break and hold carbon razor blade for single use.

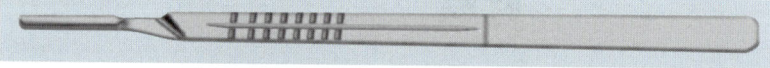

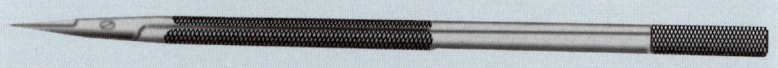

Swiss model, blade breaker

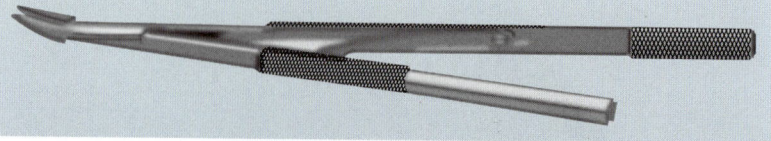

Troutman micro blade holder

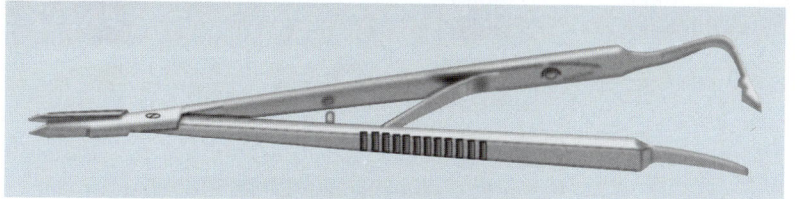

Barraquer blade holder

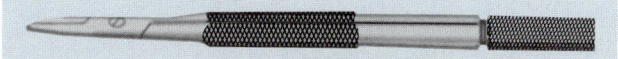

Castroviejo blade breaker and holder, small

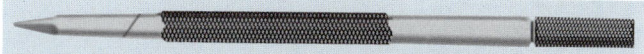

Castroviejo blade breaker and holder, big

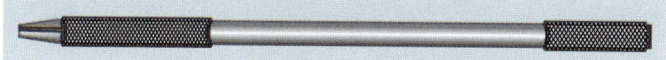

Chuck handle

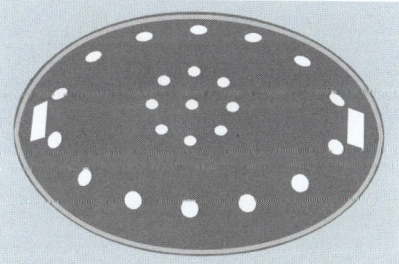

Eye shield

Cataract Knife

• Cutting out of the anterior chamber from the inside through the limbus.

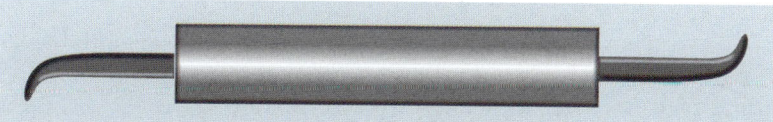

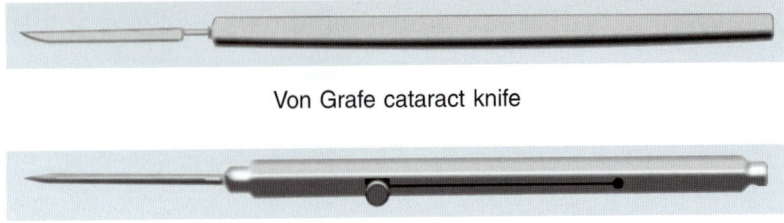

Von Grafe cataract knife

Barraquer cataract knife in sliding case

Discission Knife

• Used to do the needling for congenital cataract.

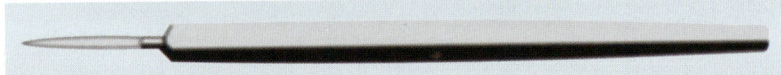

Zeigler's Knife

• Very tiny knife for intraocular manoeuvres specially when space is less.

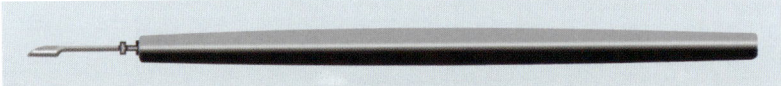

Keratotome

Diamond-shaped blade with a sharp apex and two cutting edges.

Uses

• Valvular corneal incisions for entry into the anterior chamber for all modern techniques of cataract extraction.
• Self-sealing incisions for phacoemulsification and manual SICS operation.

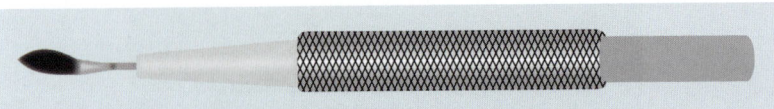

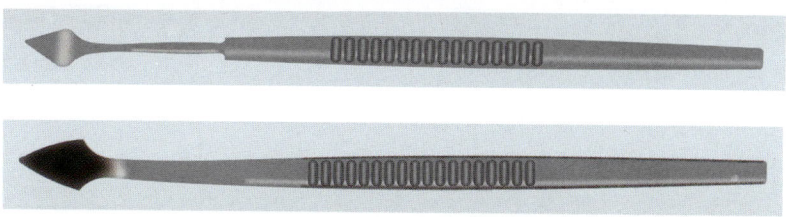

Lamellar Dissector Knives

- Making sclerocorneal tunnels in keratoplasty and small incision cataract surgery (SICS).
- For partial splitting of cornea/sclera.

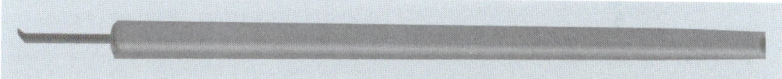

Paufique graft knife angled tip, curve cutting edge

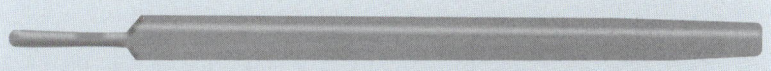

Tooke corneal knife straight blade with curved cutting edge

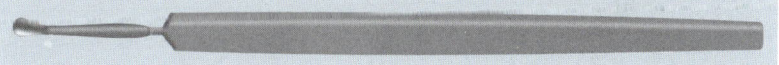

Gill corneal knife with curved cutting edge

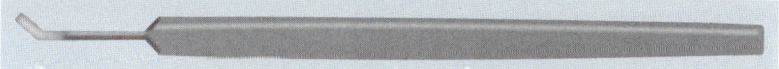

Paton's corneal dissector, hockey stick knife

Other Knives

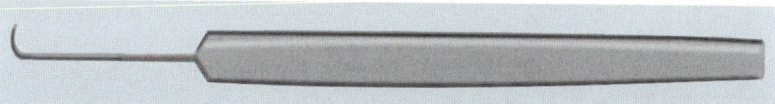

Emery cystitome with cutting edge, for push and pull cutting

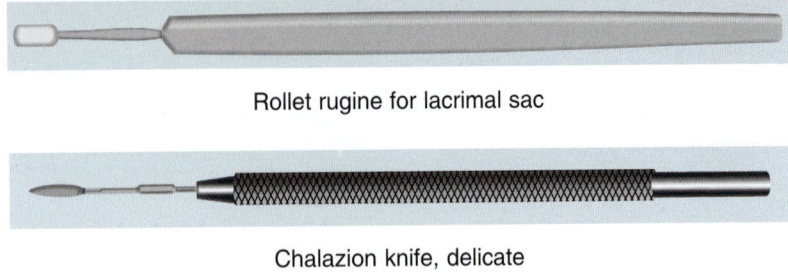

Rollet rugine for lacrimal sac

Chalazion knife, delicate

Micro round knife with visco canalostome

Diamond Knife

• Used to perform microincisions on the cornea during radial kerato-tomy.

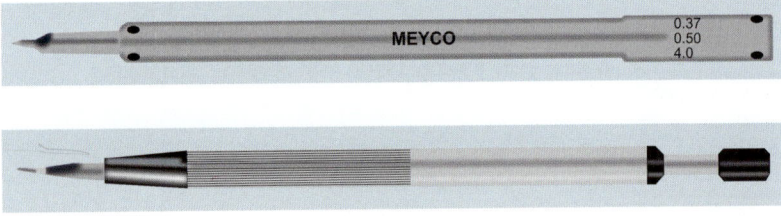

Rougine

• A rougine is an instrument used in conjunctival/sac surgery.

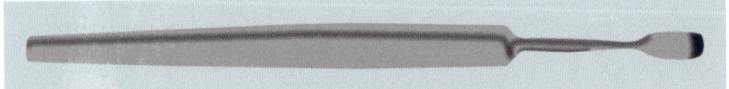

Side Port Entry Blade

• Straight knife with a sharp pointed tip and cutting on one side.

Uses

- It is used to make a small valvular clear corneal incision (commonly called as side port incision) in phacoemulsification and other intra-ocular surgeries including pars plana vitrectomy.

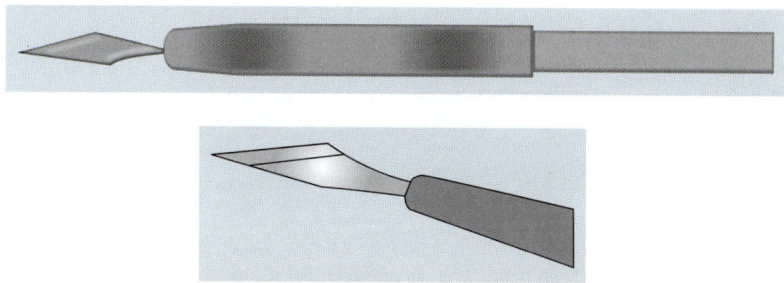

Crescent Knife (Sclerocorneal Splitter)

Blunt-tipped, bevel up knife having cut-splitting action at the tip and both the sides.

Uses

- It is used to make tunnel incision in the sclera and cornea for phaco-emulsification, manual small incision cataract surgery (SICS), and trabeculectomy.
- Making sclerocorneal tunnels in "small incision cataract surgery".
- For scleral lamellar dissection in glaucoma surgery.
- For corneal lamellar dissection in lamellar keratoplasty.

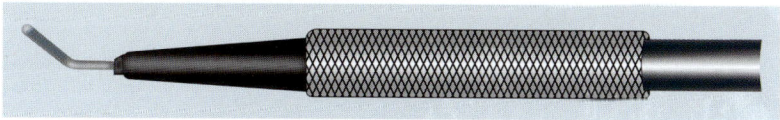

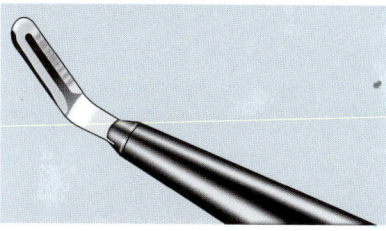

NEEDLE HOLDER

- Holding the needle in position while applying sutures.
- Silcock's needle holder has a catch and is used for heavier gauge needles.
- Used mainly for skin, muscle and corneal incisions.

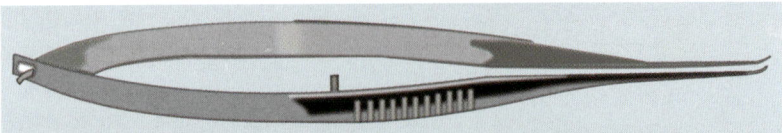

Arruga's Needle Holder

- Has a catch (lock) and is used for heavier gauge needles (thicker than 6-0).
- Used mainly for skin and muscle incisions.

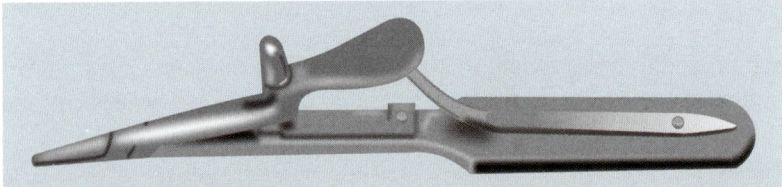

Other Heavy Needle Holders

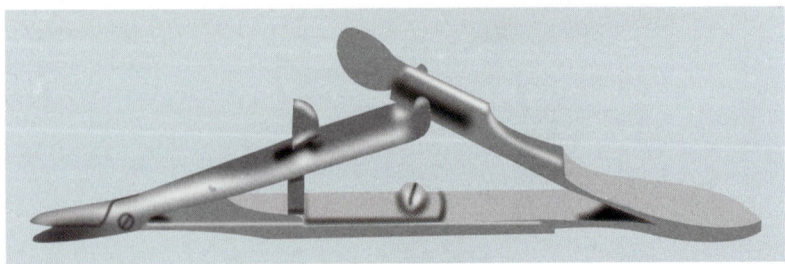

Kalt needle holder

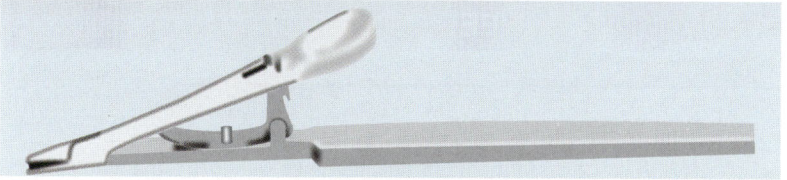

Silcock needle holder

Barraquer's Needle Holder

- Small instrument with a spring action with or without a catch used for finer gauge needles (5-0 or finer).
- Used mainly to suture intraocular and corneal incisions.

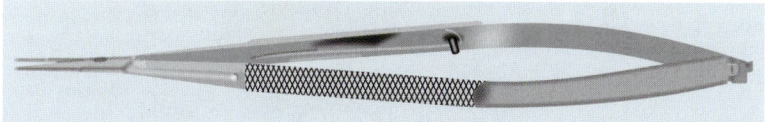

Barraquer needle holder, very delicate jaws, straight

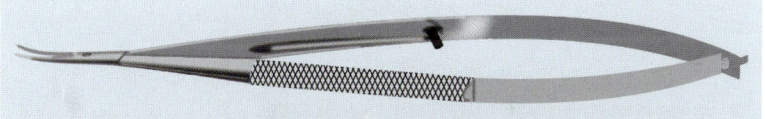

Barraquer needle holder, very delicate jaws, curved

Other Fine Needle Holders

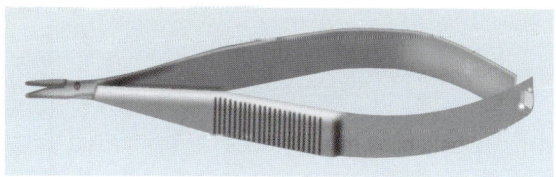

Castroviejo needle holder, delicate jaws with lock, straight

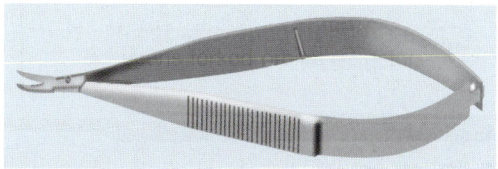

Castroviejo needle holder, delicate jaws with lock, curved

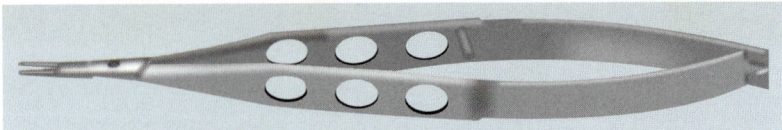

McPherson needle holder, delicate jaws with lock, straight

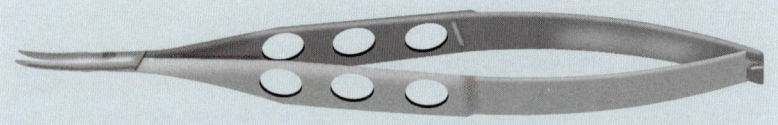

McPherson needle holder, delicate jaws with lock, curved

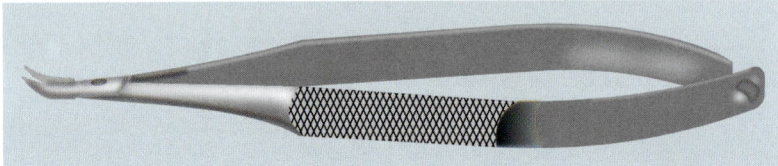

Troutman needle holder, delicate strongly curved jaws, without lock

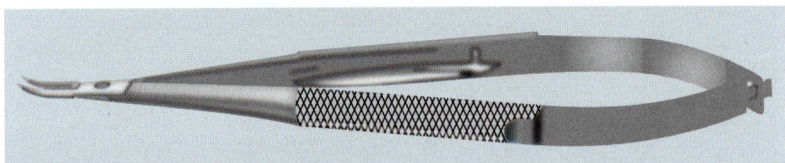

Anis needle holder, extra delicate jaws

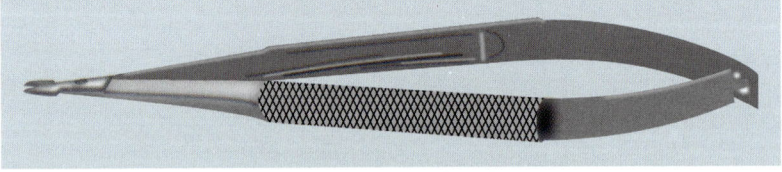

McIntyre fish hook needle holder

Hooks, Spatula and Lens Expresser

- To hold the muscle.
- To express the nucleus.
- To retract the pupil.

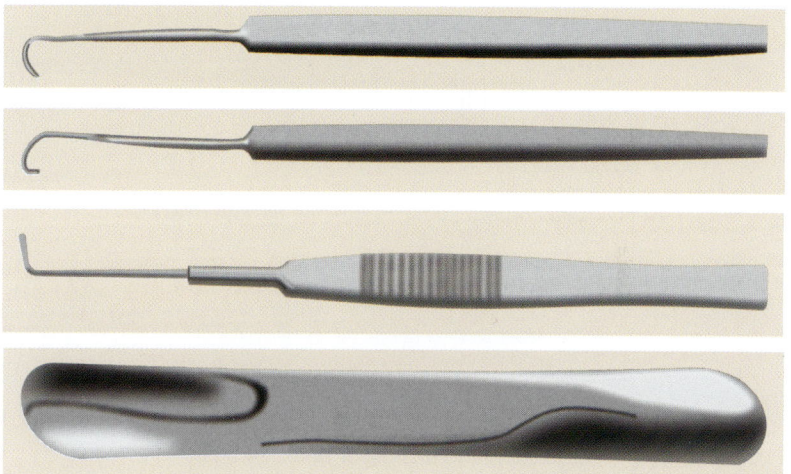

Muscle (Strabismus) Hook

It is similar to the lens expressor in appearance but has a blunt gurding knob at the end to prevent muscle slippage. The plane of the handle is the same as that of the curvature of the hook.

Uses

1. To engage the extraocular muscles during surgery for squint, enucleation, and retinal detachment.
2. In the absence of lens expressor, it may be used in its place.

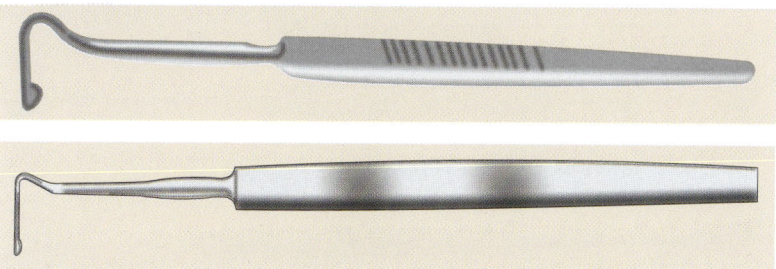

Muscle hook, 14 cm

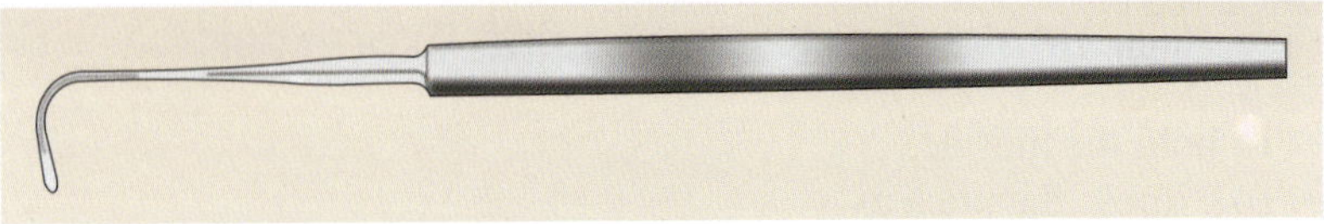

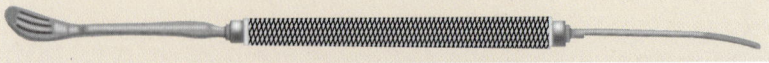

Strabismus hook, 14 cm

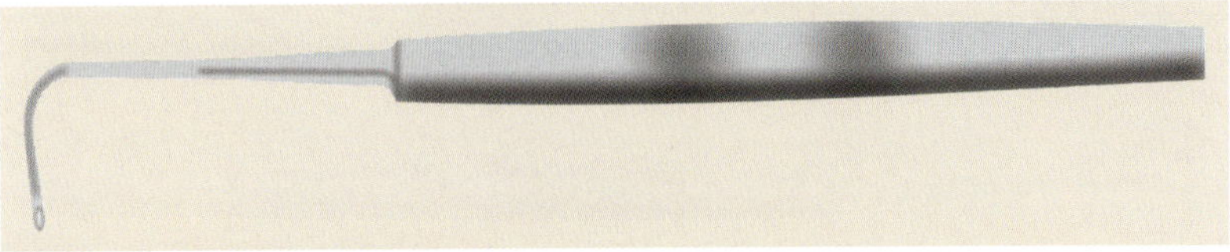

Retinal detachment hook, 14 cm, flat tip with oval hole

Lens Loop with Hook

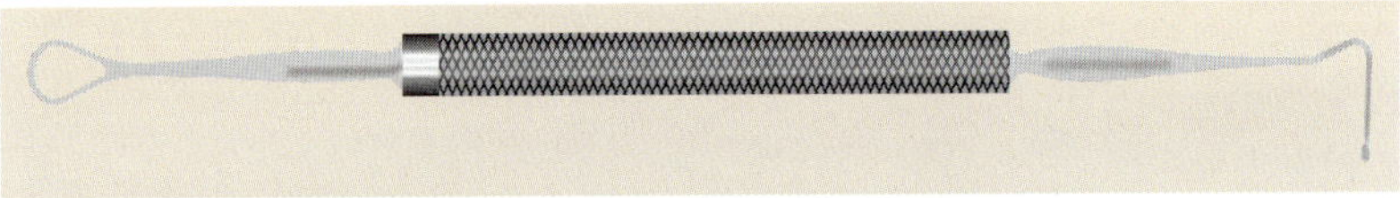

Lens loop and expressor hook, 14.5 cm

Spatula

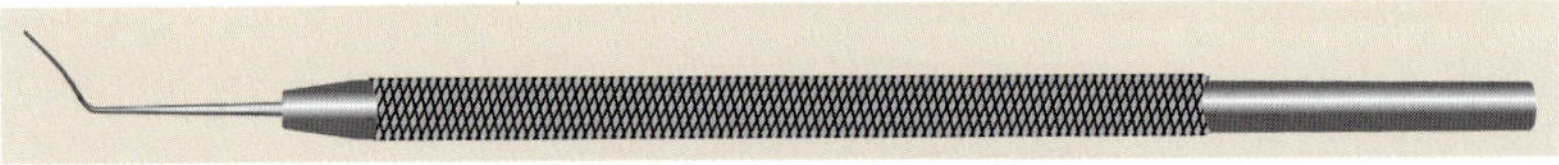

Castroviejo cyclodialysis spatula

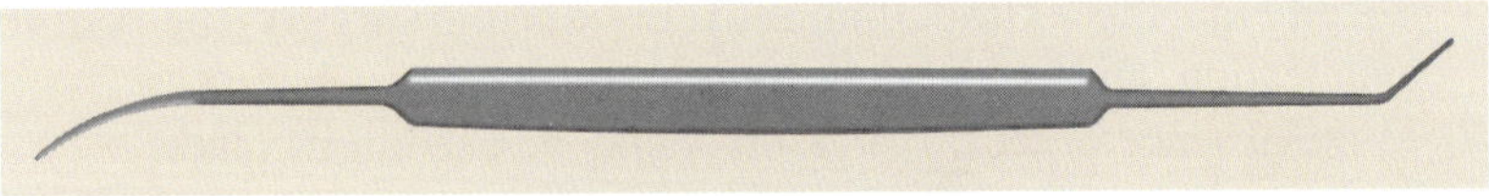

Koman Nair iris spatula

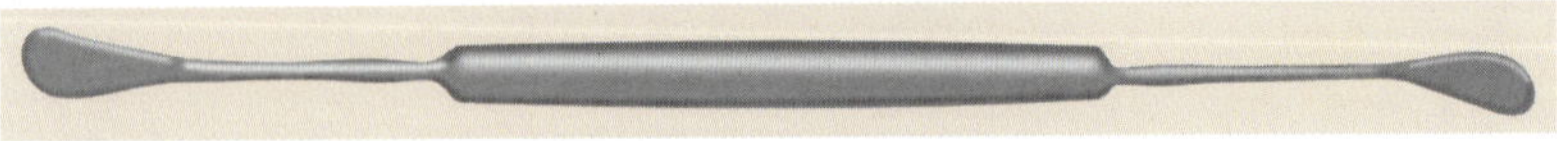

Green lens spatula

Grafe lens spatula

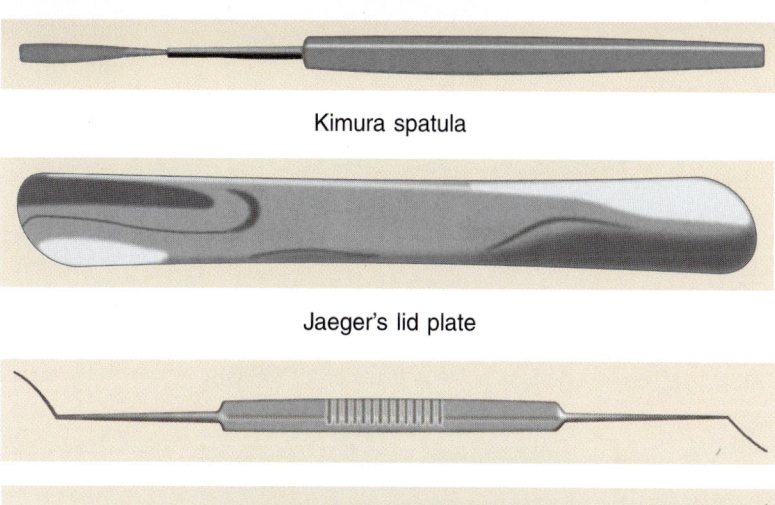

Kimura spatula

Jaeger's lid plate

Castroviejo cyclodialysis spatula

Iris Repositor

Handle with blade and blunt end.

Uses

- To reposit iris in AC after intraocular surgery.
- To break synechiae at pupillary margin.
- To break anterior synechia.

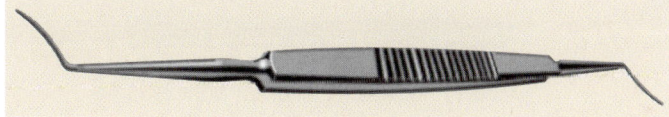

Foreign Body Spud and Needle

Spud to remove superficial and needle for the deep foreign bodies in the eye.

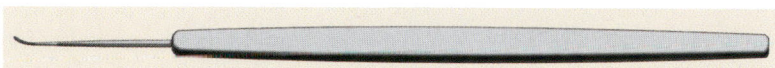

Nucleotomy Devices

Kansas nucleus bisector for MSICS

Kansas nucleus trisector for MSICS

Alfonso nucleus trisector for MSICS

Ravisankar nucleus trisector for MSICS

McIntyre nucleus bisector for MSICS

McIntyre nucleus trisector for MSICS

CHOPPERS

- It resembles Sinskey hook in shape.
- The inner edge of the bent tip is cutting and may have different angles.

Uses

It is used to split or chop the nucleus into smaller pieces and also for nuclear manipulation in phacoemulsification surgery.

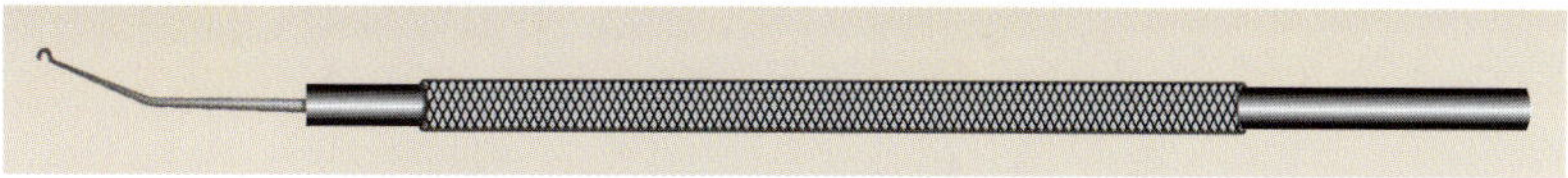

Chang micro finger phaco chopper

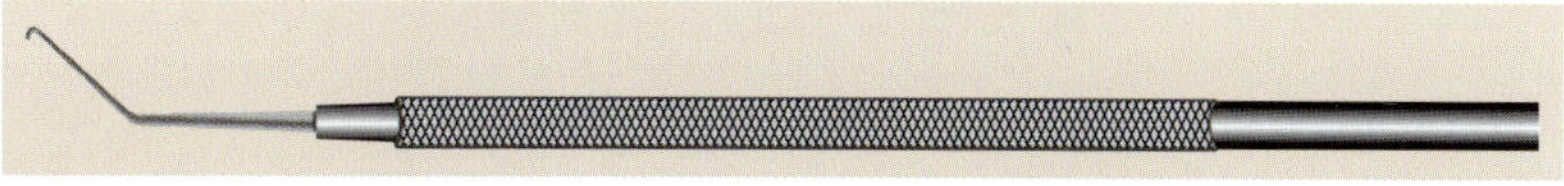

Mohan Rajan micro combo phaco chopper

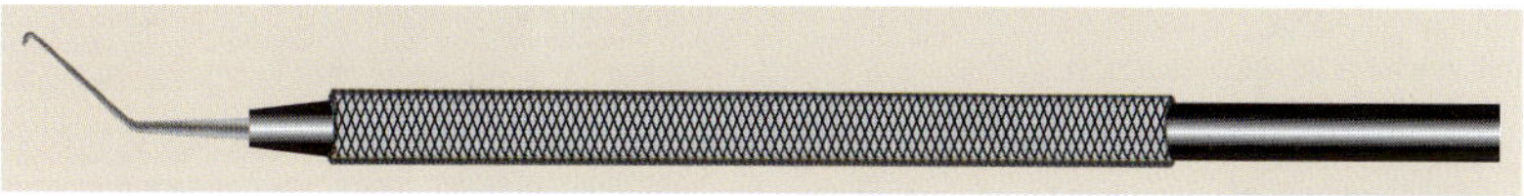

Arul phaco chopper

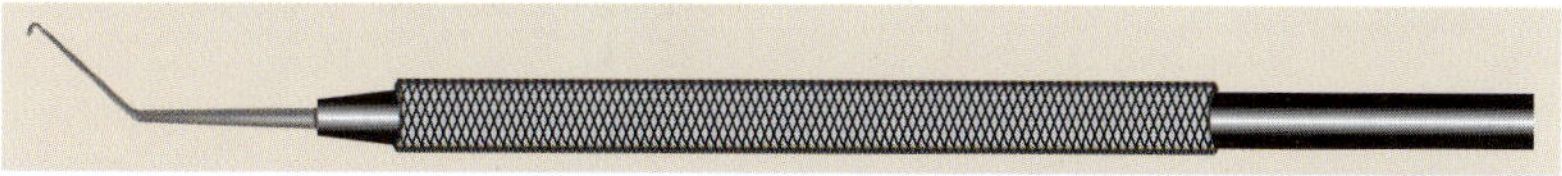

Agarwal phaco chopper

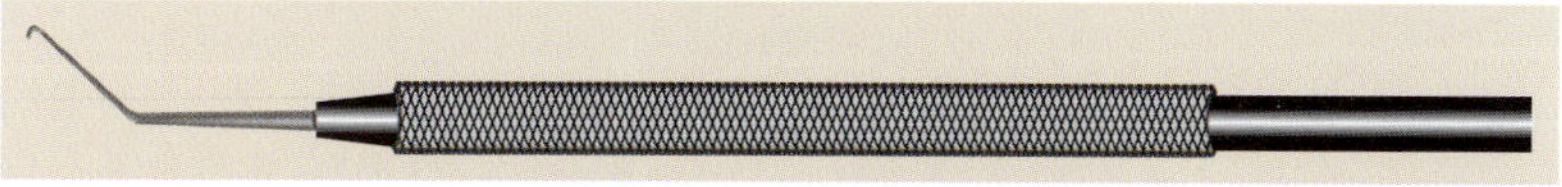

Appasamy phaco chopper

IOL

Prosthetic lenses implanted after lens removal.

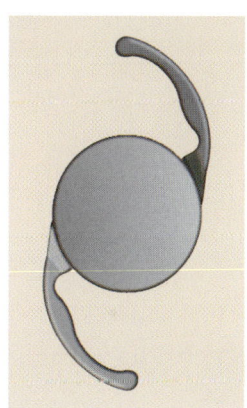 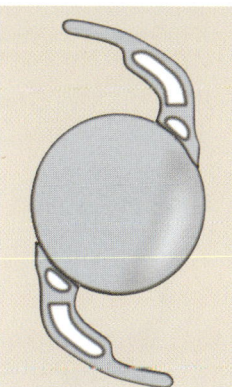 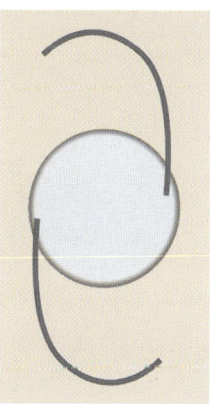

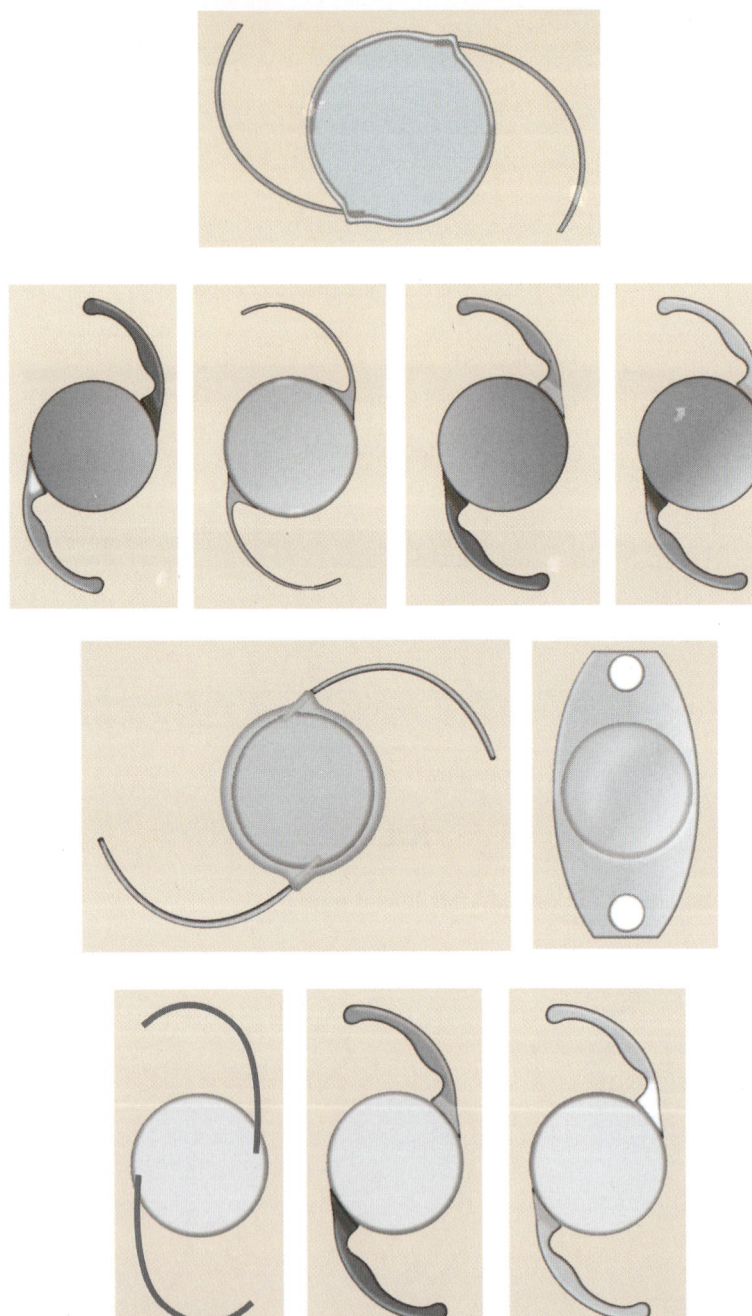

Manipulator

Angulated round hook with a handle used in manipulation/rotation of an IOL.

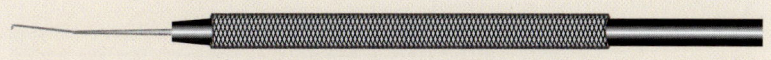

Maloney IOL manipulator

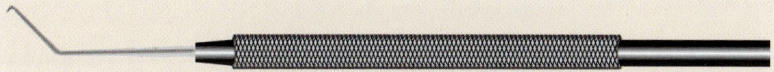

Akahoshi pre-chopper

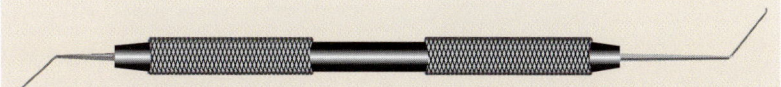

Agarwal-Bechert double edge cutter with fully cutting edge and Y manipulator

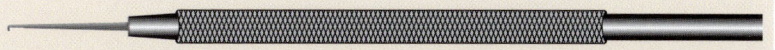

Sinskey II lens manipulating hook, blunt tip

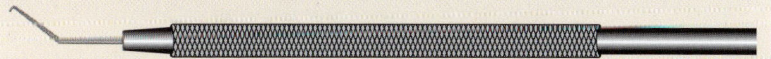

Sinskey II, straight, lens manipulating hook, blunt tip, angled

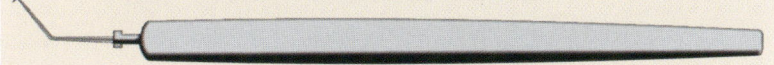

Harris lens manipulating hook, blunt tip

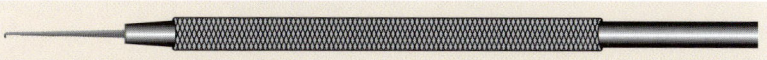

Osher Y hook no hole lens manipulator

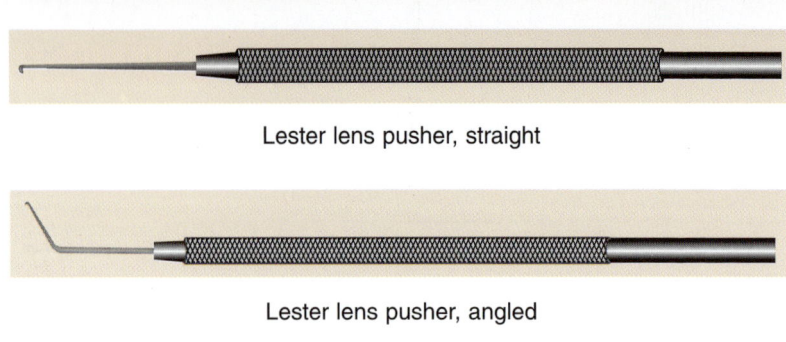

Lester lens pusher, straight

Lester lens pusher, angled

Lester no hole IOL manipulator

Lens Expressers

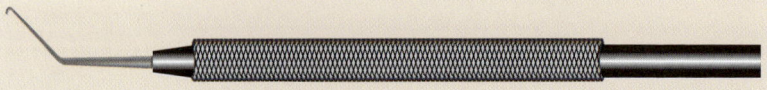

Kirby lens expresser and repositer

Kirby iris expresser and repositer

Kirby lens expresser and vectis

Capsule Polishers

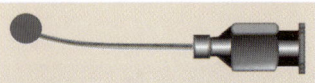

Kraff posterior capsule polishing curette, 25 gauge, with sharp irrigating port in the centre of cup .

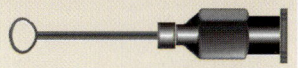

Drew's posterior capsule polisher, 25 gauge, angled ring port

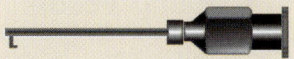

Graether collar button polisher, 23 gauge

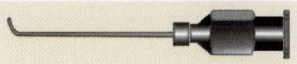

Kratzr posterior capsule scratcher, 23 gauge

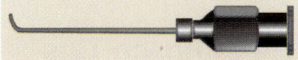

Rubman Katzin posterior capsule polisher, 22 gauge

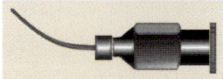

Shapiro posterior capsule polisher, 23 gauge

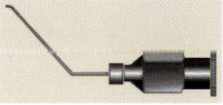

Simcoe anterior capsule polisher, 23 gauge

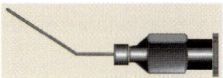

Simcoe posterior capsule polisher, 23 gauge, 45 degree angled

Vectis

It is wire loop attached to a metallic handle.

Uses

- It is used to remove dislocated or subluxated lens and nucleus in ECCE.

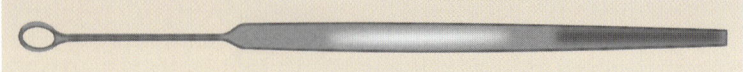

Irrigating Vectis

For nucleus delivery during MSICS.

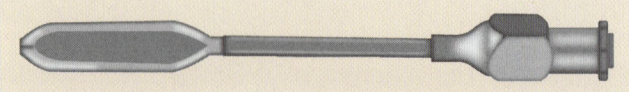

McIntyre nucleus removal spoon with irrigating ports

For Phaco Tips

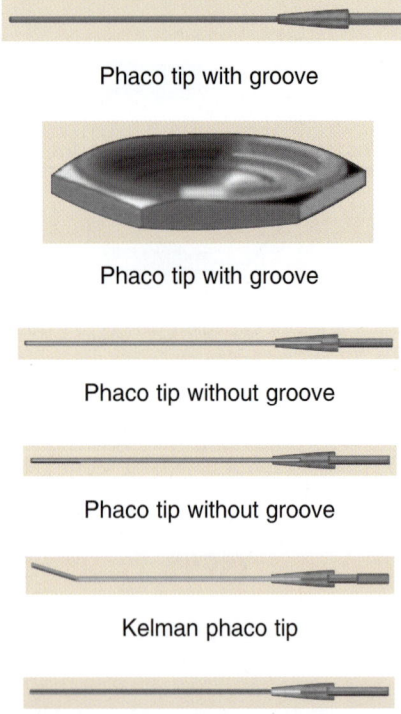

Phaco tip with groove

Phaco tip with groove

Phaco tip without groove

Phaco tip without groove

Kelman phaco tip

Phaco tip with groove for phaconit

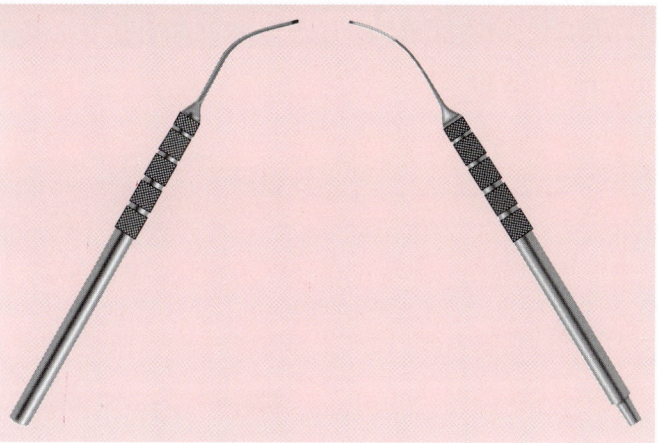

Bimanual cannula

Sinsky's Hook/IOL Dialler

Uses

1. It is used to dial the PMMA non-foldable IOL for proper positioning in the capsular bag or ciliary sulcus.
2. It can also be used to manipulate the nucleus in phacoemulsification surgery.

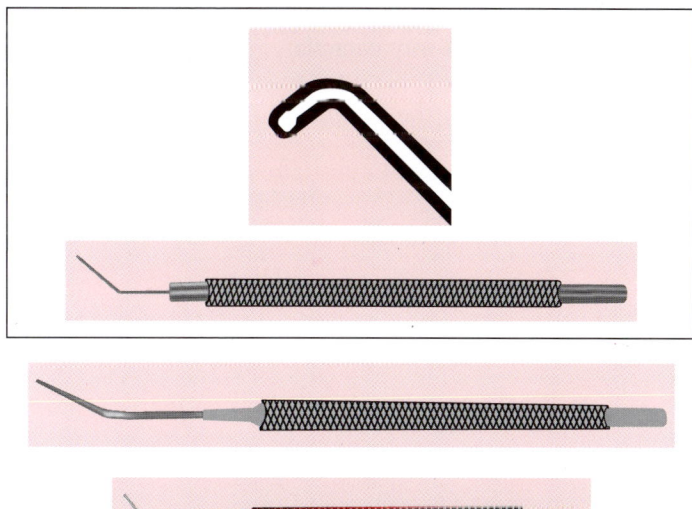

CANNULA

Used to carry fluid/air.

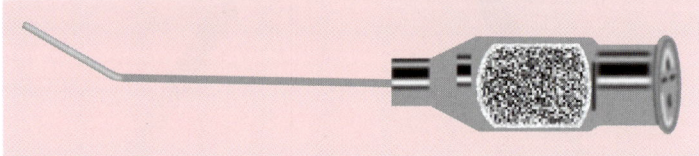

Air cannula

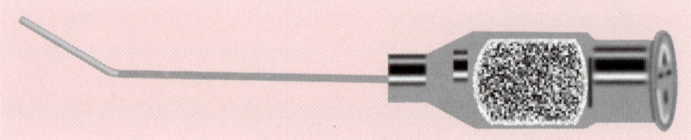

Hydro cannula

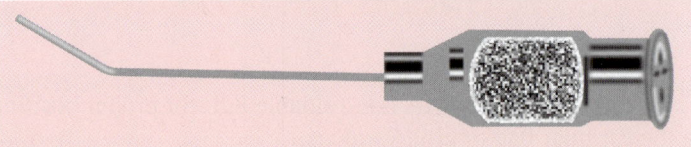

I/A Cannula

- Irrigation-aspiration two-way cannula.
- Effectively two small cannulae fitted together, one to introduce fluid and the other to extract the cortical materials, blood, etc. in eye operations.

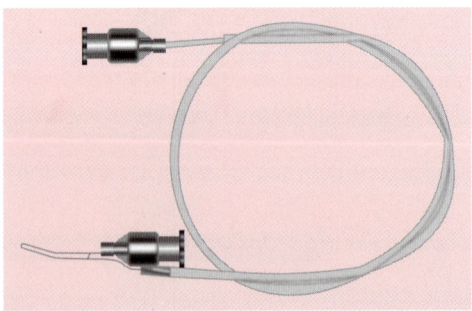

Simcoe I/A cannula, original model (direct) aspiration through silicon tube and irrigation through main hub

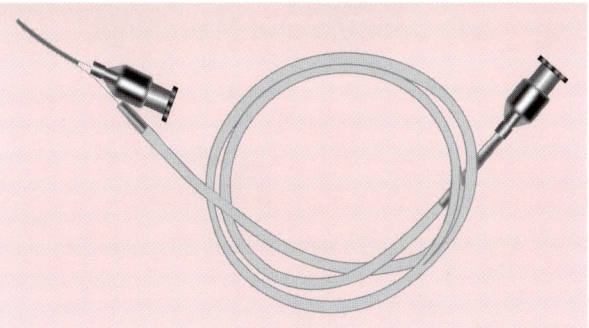

Reverse Simcoe I/A cannula, original model irrigation through silicon tube and aspiration through main hub

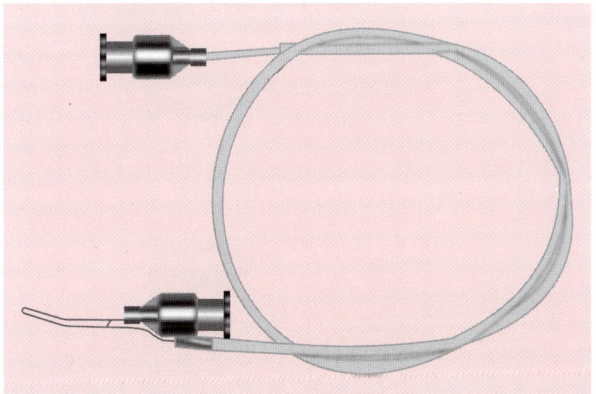

Swiss I/A cannula, aspiration through silicon tube and irrigation through main hub

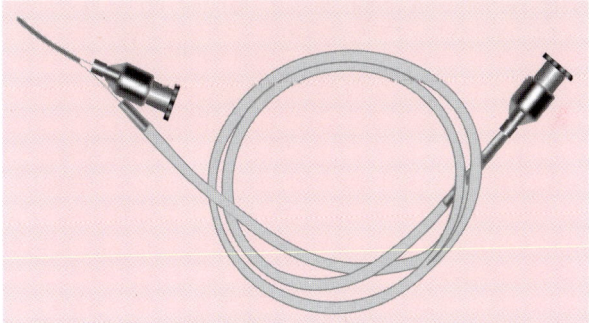

Swiss I/A cannula, aspiration through silicon tube and irrigation through main hub

A/C Cannula and Maintainer

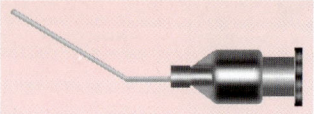

McIntyre A/C cannula, 45 degree angled, 30 gauge with blunt tip

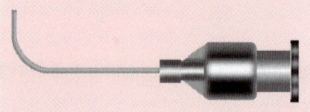

A/C cannula, 90 degree curve with 27 gauge blunt tip

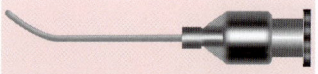

Braken A/C cannula, flattened bevelled tip

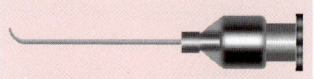

Knolle A/C cannula, 45 degree angled

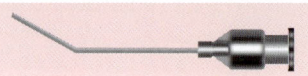

Bishop Harmon A/C cannula, flat, blunt tip, 40 degree angled

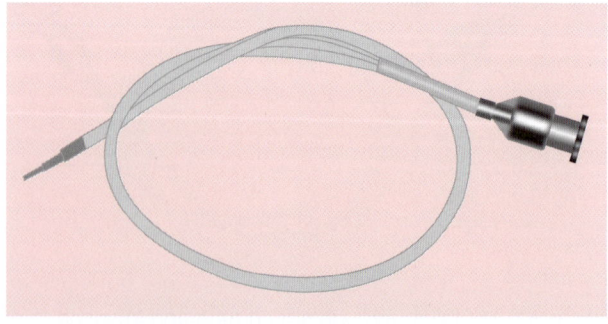

Lewicky A/C maintainer, 20 gauge

Hydro-dissection Cannula

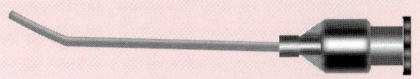

Blumenthal hydro-dissection cannula

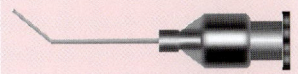

Blumenthal irrigation cystitome

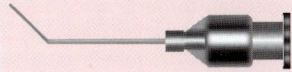

Pearce hydro-dissection cannula, 35 degree angled, blunt tip

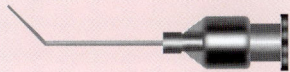

Rainin air injection cannula, spatulated, blunt tip

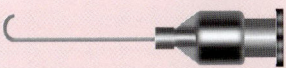

Gimbel U-shaped hydro-dissection cannula

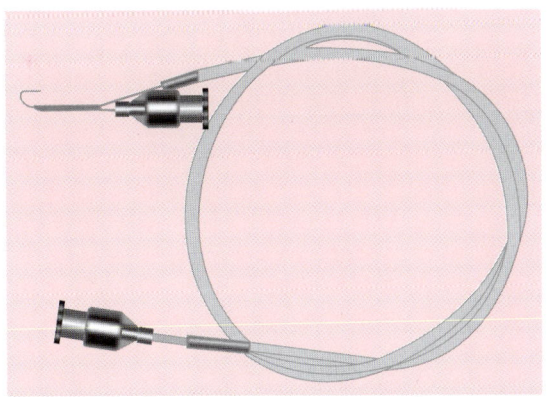

J-shaped I/A cannula, aspiration through silicon tube and irrigation through main hub, left (To aspirate 12 O'clock lens matter)

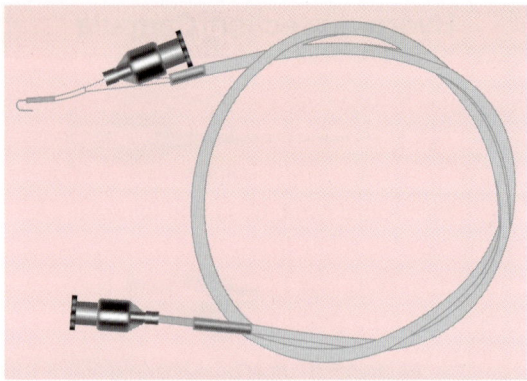

J-shaped I/A cannula, aspiration through silicon tube and irrigation through main hub, right (To aspirate 12 O'clock lens matter)

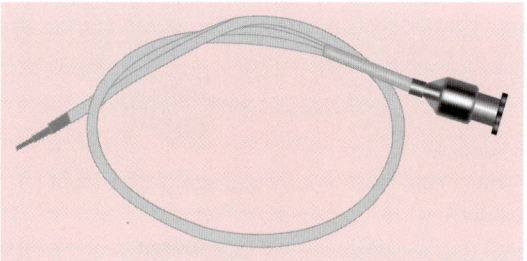

Ruit I/A cannula, aspiration through silicon tube and irrigation through main hub, original model

SCOOP & SPOON

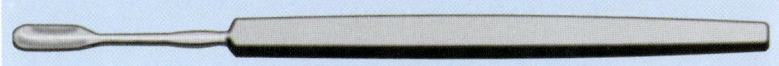

Daviel lens spoon

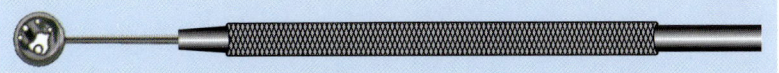

Barraquer lenticular spoon for corneal donor button transfer

Chalazion Scoop & Spoon

To remove the granulation tissue from a chalazion during surgery.

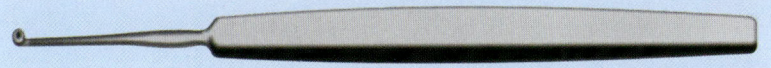

Meyerthoefer chalazion scoop, Size 0

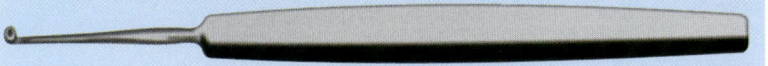

Meyerthoefer chalazion scoop, Size 1

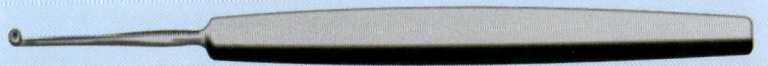

Meyerthoefer chalazion scoop, Size 2

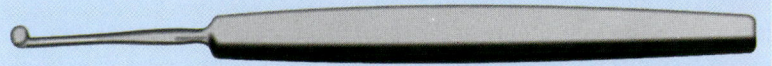

Meyerthoefer chalazion scoop, Size 3

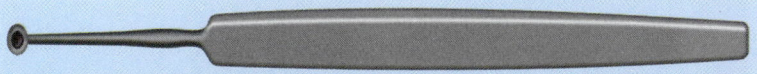

Meyerthoefer chalazion scoop, Size 4

Optic Nerve Guide (Enucleation Spoon)

It is a spoon-shaped instrument with a central cleavage.

Use

To engage the optic nerve during enucleation.

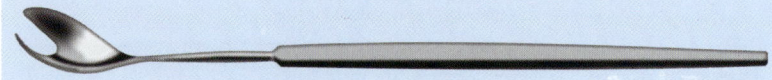

Well's enucleation scoop

Evisceration Curette

It consists of an oval or rounded shallow cup with blunt margins attached to a stout handle.

Use

To curette out the intraocular contents during evisceration operation.

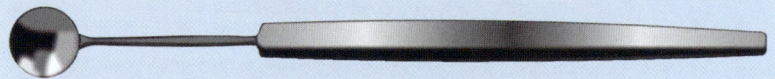

Bunge's evisceration spoon

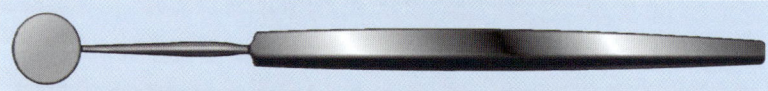

Evisceration Spoon or Scoop

Removing all the contents of the eyeball during evisceration (complete removal of all structures within the eye in diseases like endophthalmitis, traumatic disorganised globe).

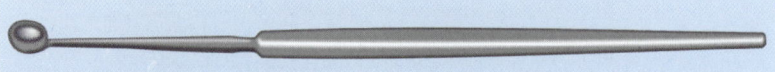

Bunge's evisceration spoon, small

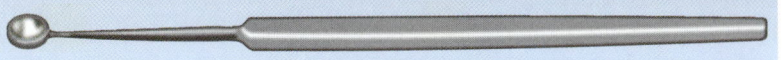

Bunge's evisceration spoon, large

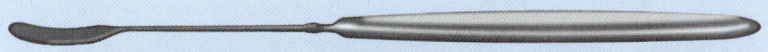

Mule evisceration scoop

Trephines and Block

Used for cutting out the cornea in a circular fashion.

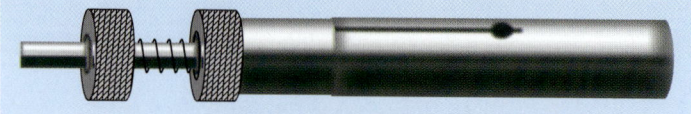

Castroviejo corneal trephine with adjustable stop

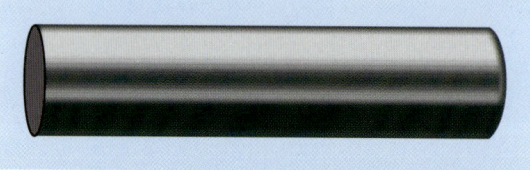

Appasamy see-through corneal trephine

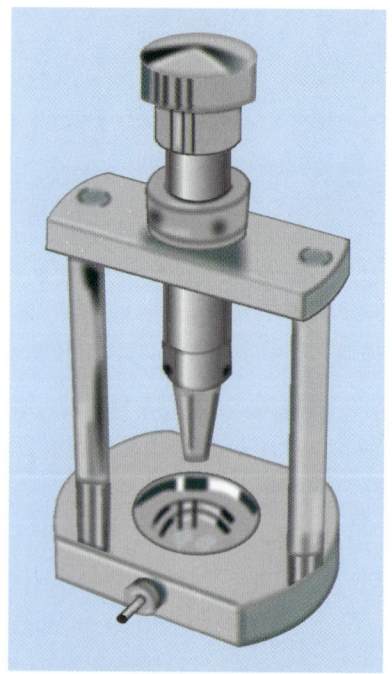

Appasamy punch trephine

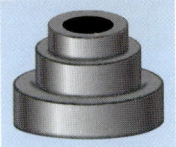

Tudor Thomas eyeball stand

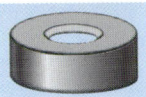

Lieberman graft cutting teflon block

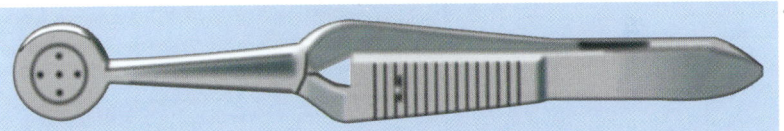

Dastoor donor corneal button holding forceps

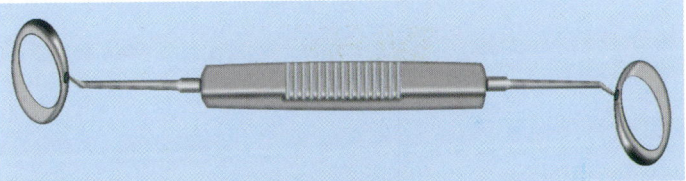

Laswk trephine

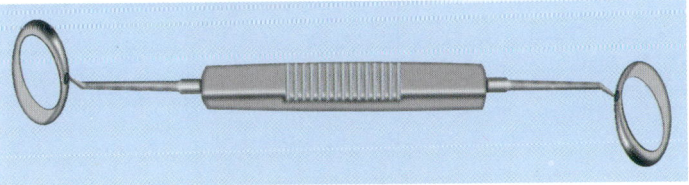

Laqsek trephine

Calipers

It is used to take measurements during squint, ptosis, retinal detachment and pars plana vitrectomy surgery. It is used to measure the pterygium size and graft size during Conjunctival Auto Graft (CAG) surgery. It is used to measure corneal diameter and visible horizontal iris diameter.

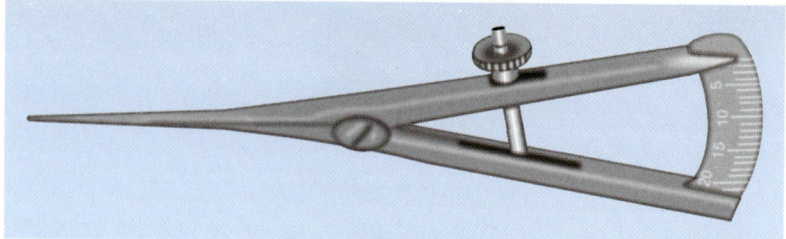

Castroviejo calliper, straight

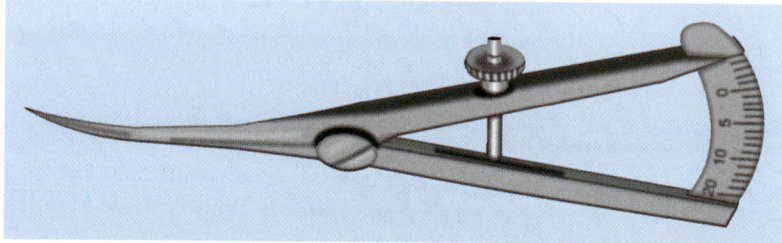

Castroviejo calliper, curved

Other Measuring Devices

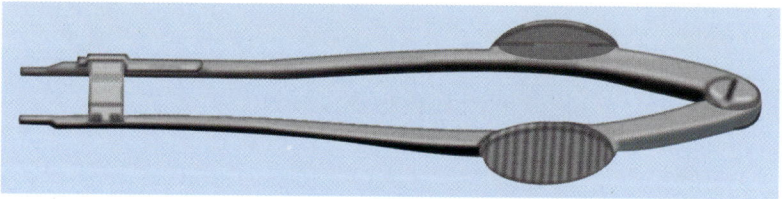

Osher calliper for internal measurement in cataract surgery

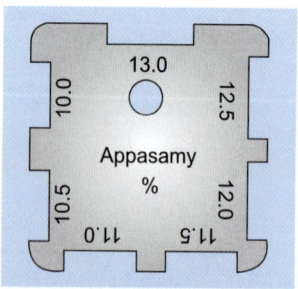

Stahl AC calliper

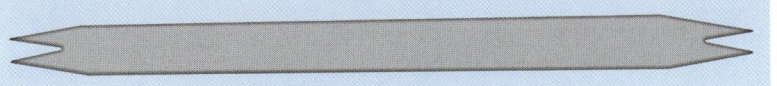

Appasamy fixed calliper, double end

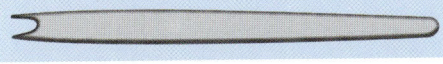

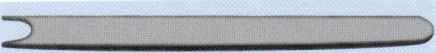

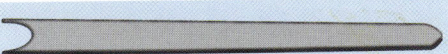

Galand incision marker

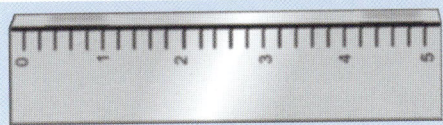

Blade gauge

Markers

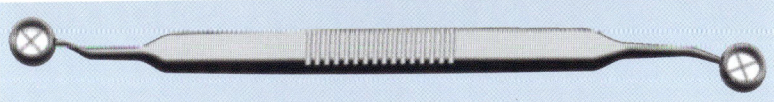

McDonald optic zone marker with cross hair

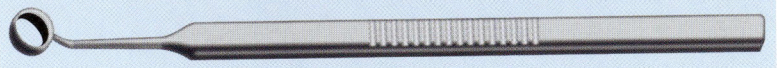

Bores optic zone marker

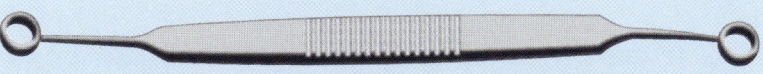

Berkley optic zone marker, double end

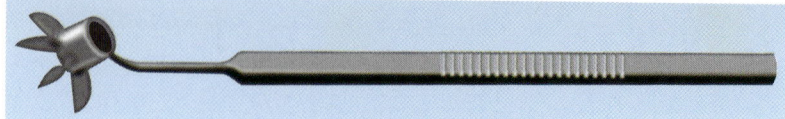

Osher Neumann RK marker with cross hair

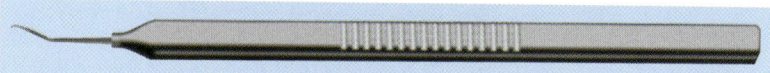

Gren visual axis marker

Toric Marker

To mark 0 to 180 degree reference mark for toric IOL implant.

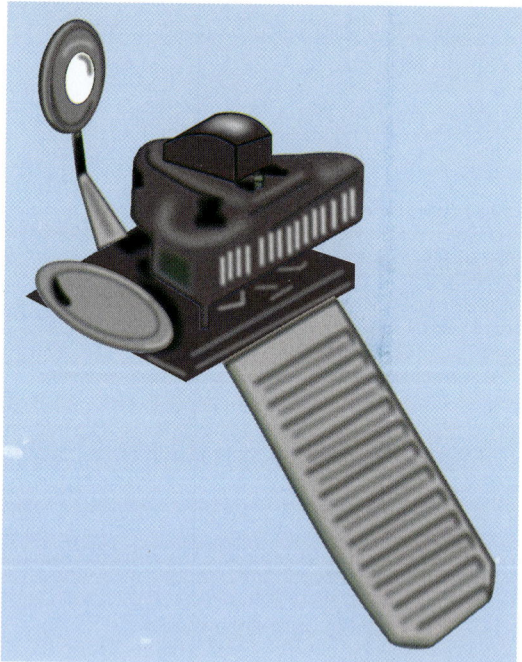

Markers and Depth Gauge

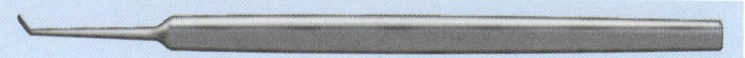

Deitz incision depth gauze for corneal incision

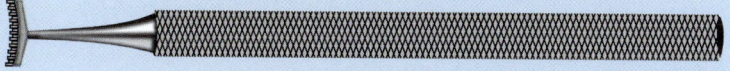

Thornton limbal incision ruler

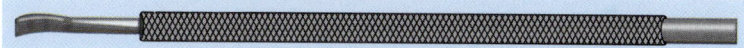

Grandon incision marker

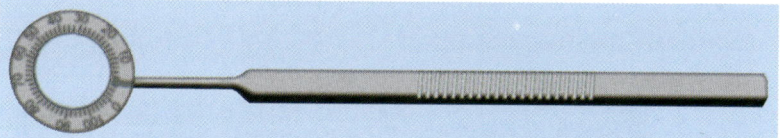

Degree gauge for accurate axial measurement

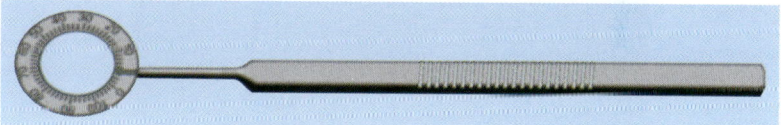

Appasamy fixation ring and degree gauge

Hams Probe (Special Instruments for Trabeculotomy)

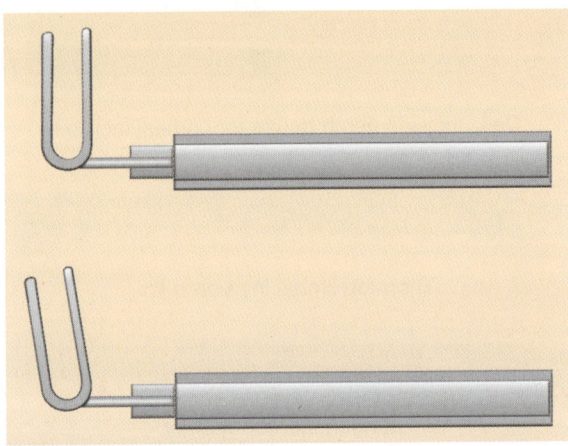

Glaucoma Valve (Special Device for Valve Surgery)

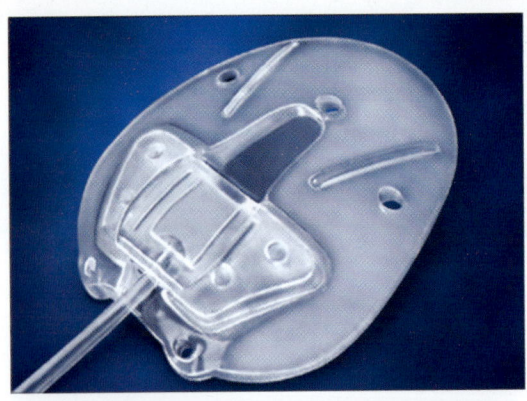

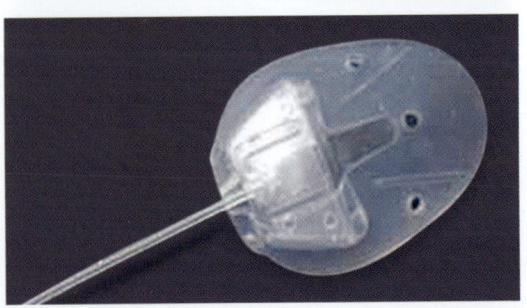

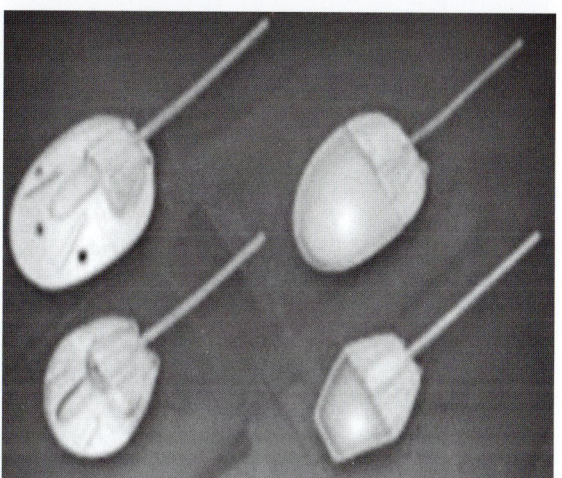

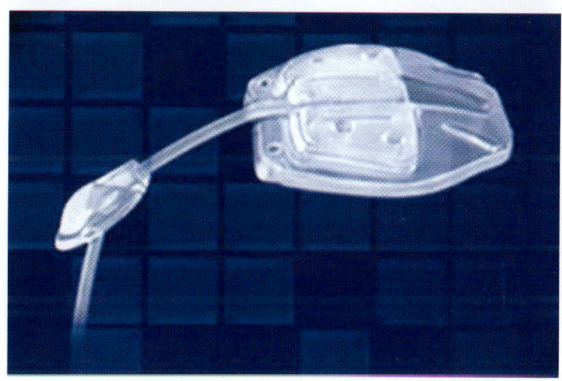

Glaucoma valve

Nasal Speculum and Nasal Forceps

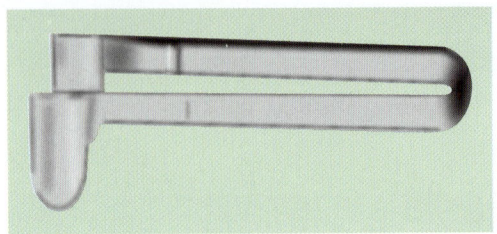

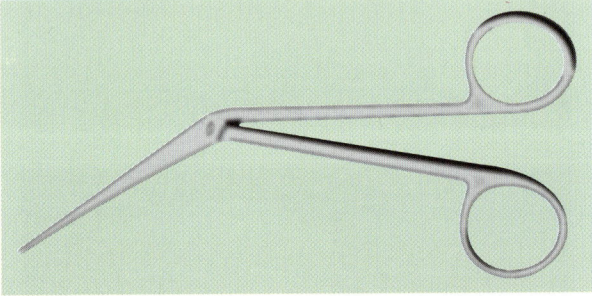

Nettleship's punctum dilator

To dilate the lacrimal punctum of the lacrimal apparatus of the eye for syringing or operations

Bowman's Lacrimal Probe

These are a set of straight metal wires of varying thickness (size 0-8) with blunt rounded ends and flattened central platform.

Uses

1. To probe nasolacrimal duct in congenital blockage.
2. To identify the lacrimal sac during DCT and DCR operations, probing the nasolacrimal duct.

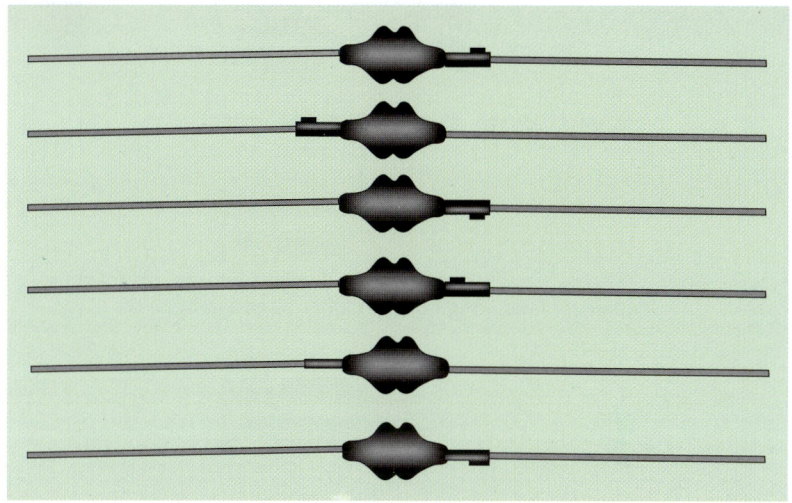

Lacrimal Cannula

Small curved cannula the size of a syringe needle used to introduce fluids or drugs into the lacrimal passage, to test its patency or during surgery (DCR).

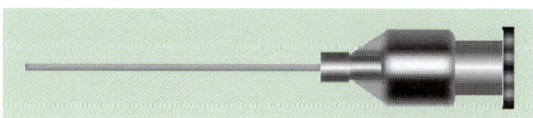

McIntyre lacrimal cannula, straight, 23 gauge blunt tip

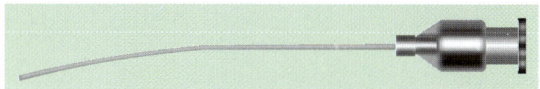

Lacrimal curved cannula, 23 gauge maleable tip

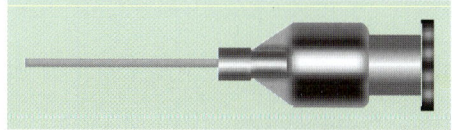

Lacrimal cannula, straight, 27 gauge maleable tip

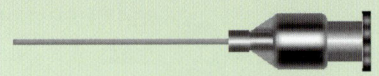

Lacrimal cannula, straight, 30 gauge maleable tip

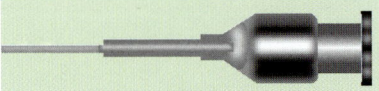

Lacrimal cannula, long hub, straight, 23 gauge blunt tip

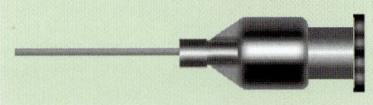

Bailey lacrimal cannula, straight, 20 gauge blunt tip

Thermocautery

- To cauterise the bleeding vessels.

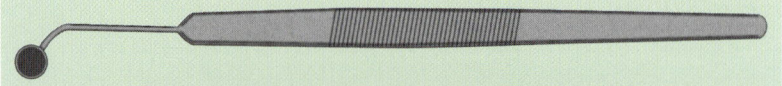

Lacrimal Dissector with Scoop

Lacrimal sac dissector and curette is a cylindrical instrument, one end of which is a blunt-tipped dissector and the other end is curetted.

Use

In lacrimal sac surgery.

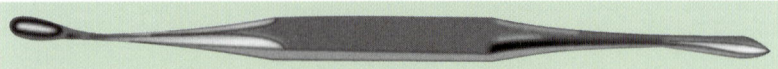

Self-Retaining Lacrimal Wound (Muller's) Retractor

- It is made up of two limbs with three curved pins on each for engaging the edges of the skin in incision.

- The limbs are kept in a retracted position with the help of a fixing screw.

Uses

- It is used to retract the skin during surgery on the lacrimal sac [e.g. dacryocystectomy (DCT) or dacryocystorhinostomy (DCR)].

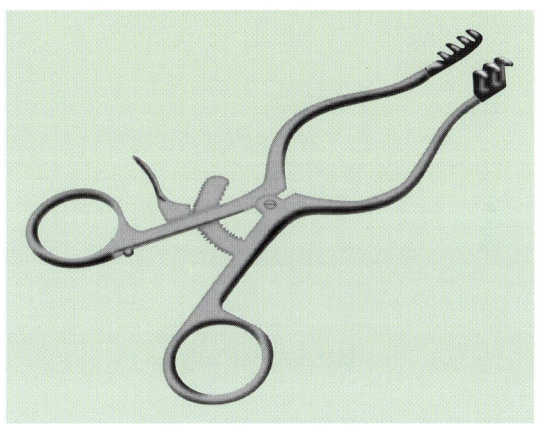

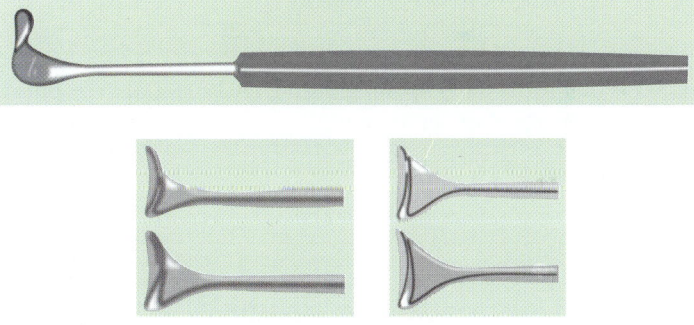

Desmarres lid retractors with solid blades

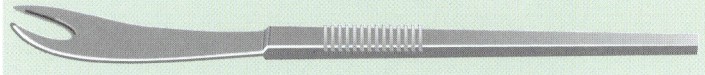

Schepens forked orbital retractor

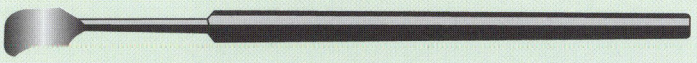

Helveston tissue retractor with thin curved blades

Hammer, Chisel and Bone Gouge

• Bone cutting and shaping.

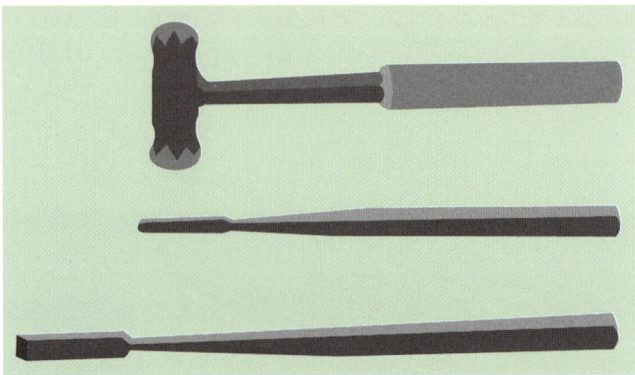

Bone Punch

To fracture pieces from a thin bone in facial surgery and during operations like dacryocystorhinostomy.

Uses

It is used to enlarge the bony opening during DCR operation by punching the bone from margins of the opening.

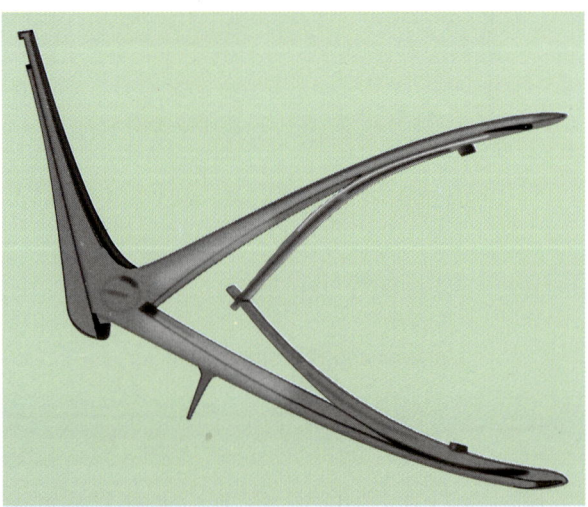

NEEDLE AND SUTURES

Suture is a material used to bring tissue together.

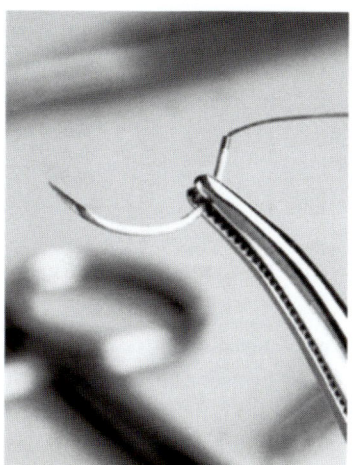

Surgical Needle

- It is rigid enough to prevent excessive bending.
- Not flexible to prevent breaking after bending.
- It is strong enough so it does not break easily.
- It is sharp enough to penetrate tissue.
- It is approximately the same diameter as the suture material; it carries to minimize trauma during passage through tissue.
- It is free of corrosion and rust to prevent infection and tissue trauma.

Basic components of the needle

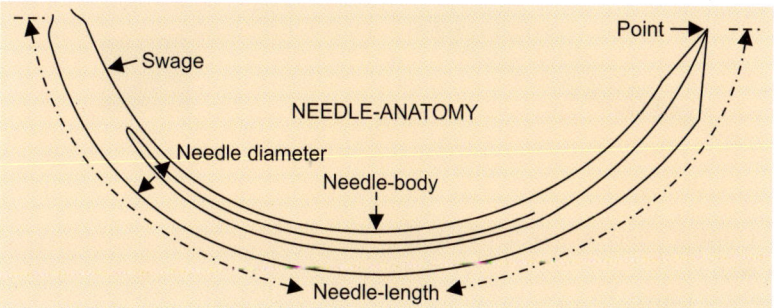

A. Points of needle

1. Cutting point: It is used to penetrate when tissue is difficult to be penetrated such as skin and tendon.
2. Reverse cutting.
3. Taper point: These needles are used in soft tissue such as intestine and peritoneum, the sharp point at the tip of needle.
4. Blunt point: These are used for suturing friable tissue such as liver and kidney.

B. Body of needle

1. Straight
2. Curved

C. Eye of the needle

The eye is the segment of needle where the suture strand is attached.
1. Eyed needle: Like any household sewing needle.
2. French eye needle: It has a slit from the inside of the eye to the end of the needle through which the suture is drawn.
3. Eyeless needle: The suture strand and the needle are one unit.

Points of needles

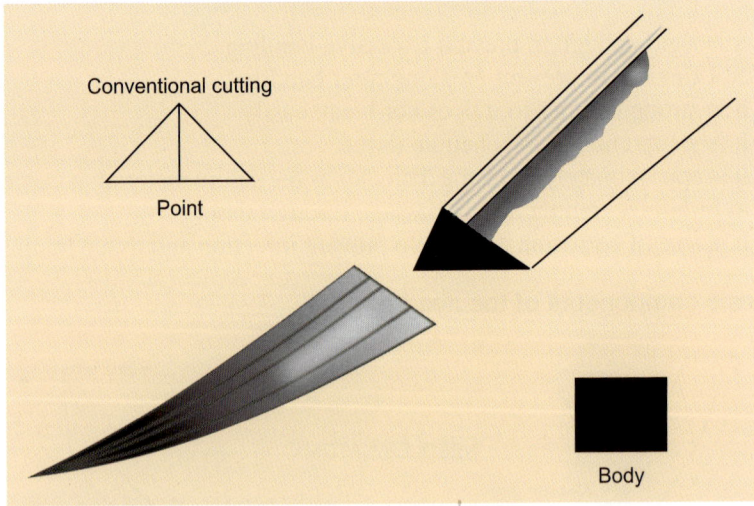

Cutting

- Cutting edge on inside of circle
- Skin
- Traumatic

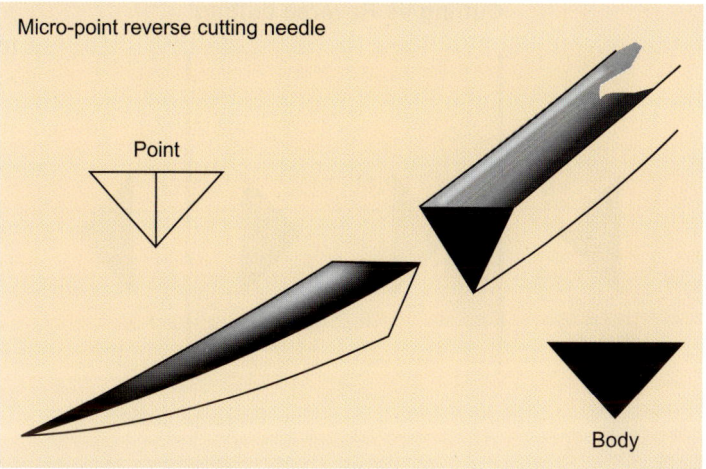

Micro-point reverse cutting needle

Point

Body

Reverse cutting

- Cutting edge on outside of circle
- Skin
- Less traumatic than cutting

Taper point

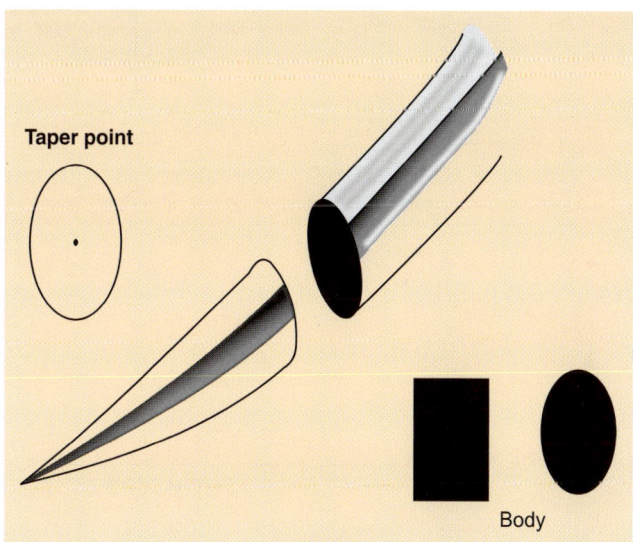

Taper point

Body

Cutting vs Reverse cutting

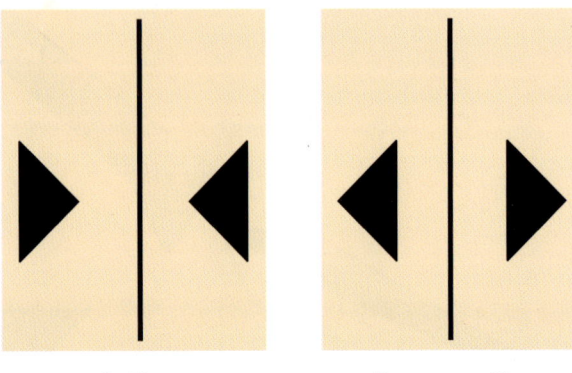

Cutting   Reverse cutting

Shapes of Needles

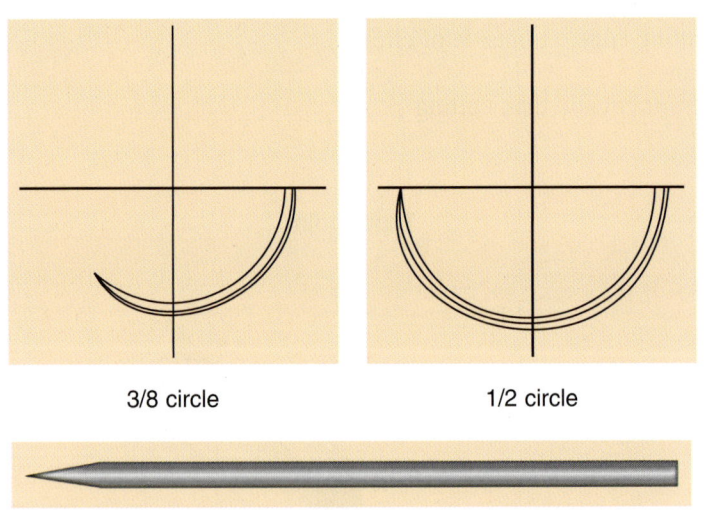

3/8 circle   1/2 circle

Straight

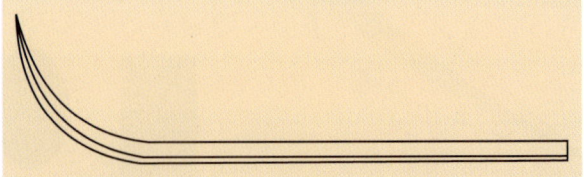

Speciality

Placement of Needle in Tissue

1. Force should always be applied in the direction that follows the curvature of the needle.

2. Suturing should always be from movable to a non-movable tissue.

3. Avoid excessive tissue bites with small needle as it will be difficult to retrieve them.

4. Use only sharp needles with minimal force. Replace dull needles.

5. Never force the needle through the tissue.

6. Grasp the needle at the body one-quarter to one-half of the length from the swaged area. Do not hold the swaged area; this may bend or break the needle. Do not grasp the point area as damage or notching may result.

7. Avoid retrieving the needle from the tissue by the tip. This will damage or dull the needle.

8. Suture should be placed in keratinized tissue whenever possible.

9. An adequate tissue bite is required to prevent the flap from tearing.

The Ideal Suture Material

- Can be used in any tissue.
- Easy to handle.
- Good knot security.
- Minimal tissue reaction.
- Unfriendly to bacteria.
- Strong yet small.
- Won't tear through tissues.
- Cheap.

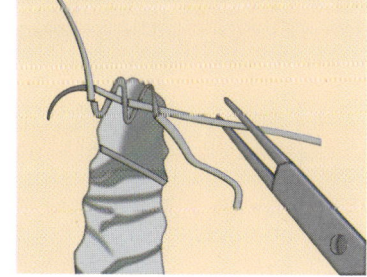

Use

To bring tissue edges together and speed wound healing.

Characteristics of Suture Material

- Absorbable vs. Non-absorbable
- Monofilament vs. Multifilament
- Natural or Synthetic

Absorbable sutures

- Internal
- Intradermal/subcuticular
- Rarely on skin

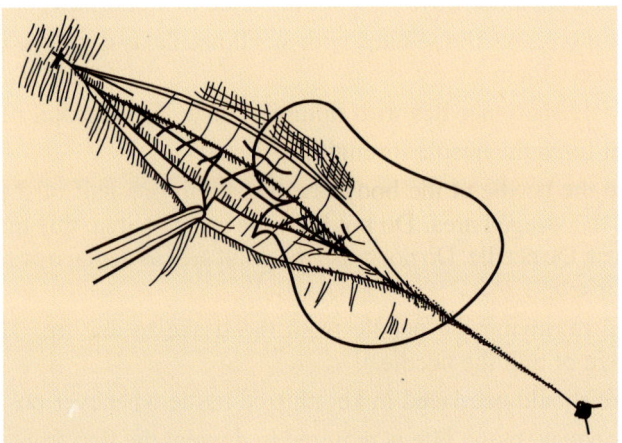

Non-absorbable suture

- Primarily skin: Needs to be removed later.
- Stainless steel = exception: Can be used internally.

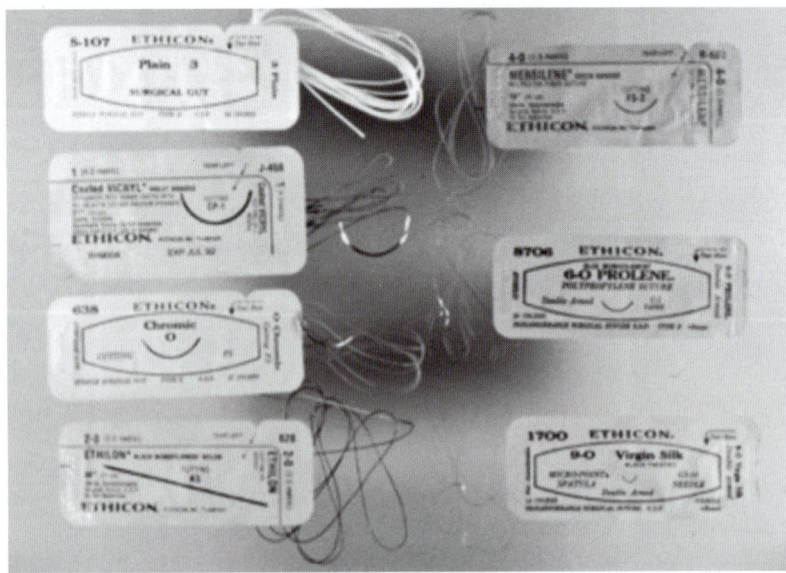

Reading the Suture Label

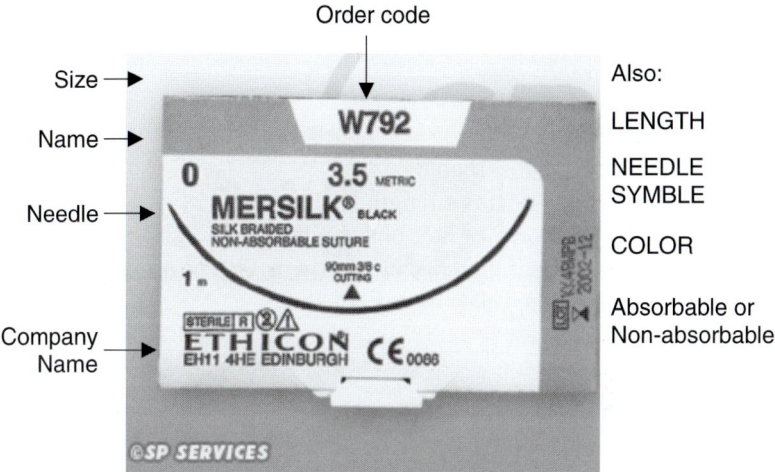

Order code

Size →

Name →

Needle →

Company Name →

Also:

LENGTH

NEEDLE SYMBLE

COLOR

Absorbable or Non-absorbable

Monofilament vs. Multifilament

Memory	Easy to handle
Less tissue drag	More tissue drag
Doesn't wick	Wicks/bacteria
Poor knot security	Good knot security
– Tissue reaction	+ Tissue reaction

Natural vs. Synthetic

- Natural
  - Gut
  - Chromic gut
  - Silk
  - Collagen
- All are absorbable

Gut/chromic gut

- Made of submucosa of small intestines.
- Multifilament.
- Breaks down by phagocytosis: inflammatory reaction common.
- Chromic: tanned, lasts longer, less reactive.
- Easy handling.
- Plain: 3–5 days.
- Chromic: 10–15 days.
- Bacteria love this stuff!

Collagen and Silk

- Natural sutures.
- VERY reactive, absorbable.
- Ophthalmic surgery only.

Vicryl (Polyglactin 910)

- Braided, synthetic, absorbable.
- Stronger than gut: Retains strength for 3 weeks.
- Broken down by enzymes, not phagocytosis.
- Breakdown products inhibit bacterial growth: Can be used in contaminated wounds, unlike other multifilaments.

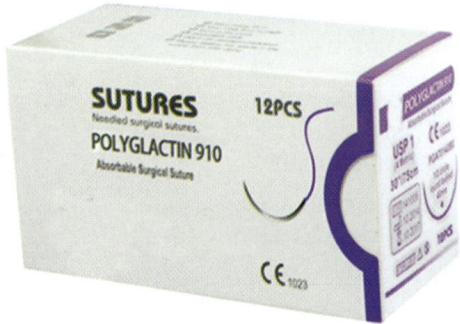

Dexon and PGA

- Polymer of glycolic acids.
- Braided, synthetic, absorbable.
- Broken down by enzymes.
- Both PGA and dexon have increased tissue drag, good knot security.
- Both are stronger than gut.

PDS (Polydioxine)

- Monofilament (less drag, worse knot security – lots of "memory").
- Synthetic, absorbable.
- Very good tensile strength (better than gut, vicryl, dexon) which lasts months.
- Absorbed completely by 182 days.

Maxon (Polyglyconate)

- Monofilament – memory.
- Synthetic, absorbable.
- Very little tissue drag.

- Poor knot security.
- Very strong.

Nonabsorbable Sutures
- Natural or Synthetic
- Monofilament or multifilament

Nylon
- Synthetic.
- Mono or Multifilament.
- Memory.
- Very little tissue reaction.
- Poor knot security.

Polymerized Caprolactum
- Vetafil, Braunamid, Supramid.
- Multifilament suture with protein coating.
- Synthetic.
- Good knot security, easy handling.
- Not very reactive.
- Don't use in contaminated wound.
- Usually comes on a reel.

Polypropylene
- Prolene, Surgilene.
- Monofilament, synthetic.
- Won't lose tensile strength over time.
- Good knot security.
- Very little tissue reaction.

Stainless Steel
- Monofilament.
- Strongest!
- Great knot security.
- Difficult handling.
- Can cut through tissues.
- Very little tissue reaction, won't harbor bacteria.

SUTURE SIZES
- Sized #5-4-3-2-1-0-00-000-0000…30-0
  – BIGGER >>>>>>>>>>>>>>>>>SMALLER

- 00 = 2-0, "two ought"
- SA : 0 through 3-0 (Optho 5-0 >>7-0)
- LA : 0 through 3
- Stainless Steel
  - In gauges (like needles)
    Smaller gauge = bigger, stronger
    Larger gauge = smaller, finer
  - 26 gauge = "ought"
  - 28 gauge = 2-0

Suture Patterns

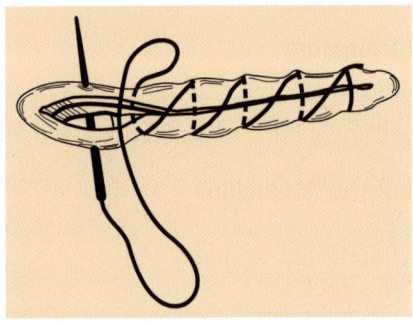

KNOT STRENGTH

- Generally 4 "throws" for > 90% knot security (nylon may need 5)
  Less "throws" = more likely to untie itself
- Stainless steel = exception again
  2 "throws" = 99% knot security

Common Suturing Techniques

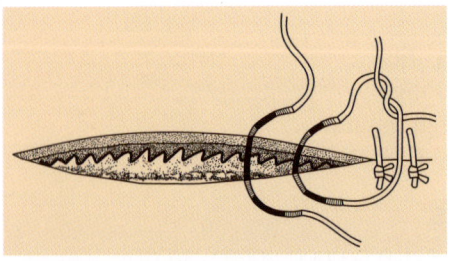

Simple Interrupted

Common Suturing Techniques (*contd.*)

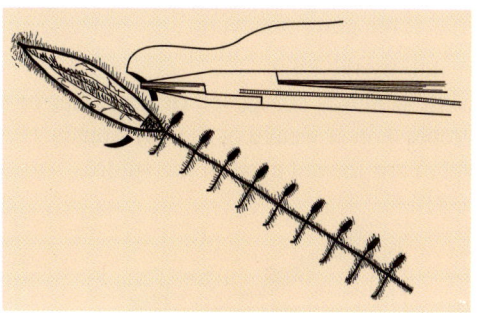

Simple Interrupted

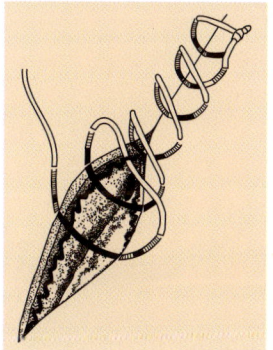

Simple continuous

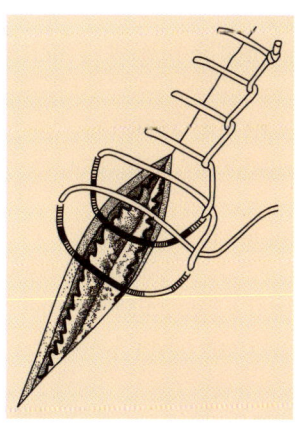

Ford interlocking

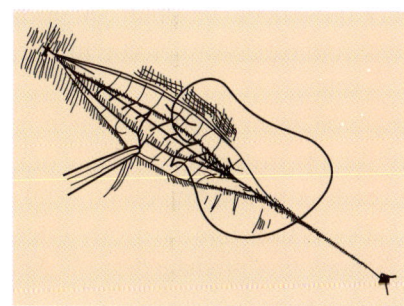

Subcuticular

Knots

A suture knot has three components:

1. The loop created by the knot.
2. The knot itself, which is composed of a number of tight "throws", each throw represents a weave of the two stands.
3. The ears, which are the cut ends of the suture.

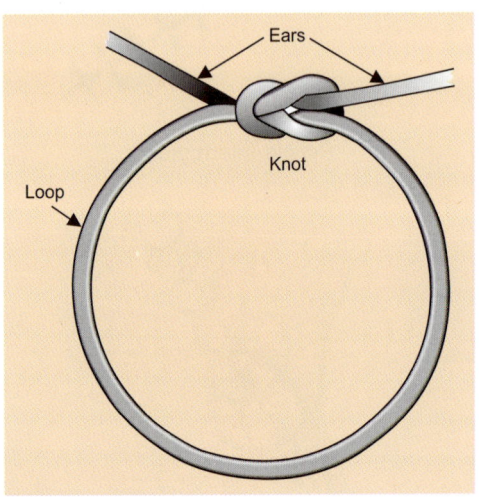

PRINCIPLES OF SUTURING

1. The completed knot must be tight, firm, and tied so that slippage will not occur.
2. To avoid wicking of bacteria, knot should not be placed in incision lines.
3. Knots should be small and the ends cut short (2–3 mm).
4. Avoid excessive tension to finer gauge materials as breakage may occur.
5. Avoid using a jerking motion, which may break the suture.
6. Avoid crushing or crimping of suture materials by not using hemostats or needle holders on them except on the free end for tying.
7. Do not tie suture too tightly as tissue necrosis may occur. Knot tension should not produce tissue blanching.
8. Maintain adequate traction on one end while tying to avoid loosening the first loop.

PRINCIPLES FOR SUTURE REMOVAL

1. The area should be swabbed with hydrogen peroxide for removal of encrusted necrotic debris, blood, and serum from about the sutures.
2. A sharp suture scissors should be used to cut the loops of individual or continuous sutures about the teeth.
3. It is often helpful to use a No. 23 explorer to help lift the sutures if they are within the sulcus or in close opposition to the tissue.
4. A cotton pliers is used to remove the suture. The location of the knots should be noted so that they can be removed first. This will prevent unnecessary entrapment under the flap.

Suture should be removed in 7 to 10 days to prevent epithelialization or wicking about the suture.

Section 2

INSTRUMENTS FOR OPHTHALMIC SURGERY (SURGERY-WISE SETS)

CATARACT

Intracapsular Cataract Extraction Set (ICCE)

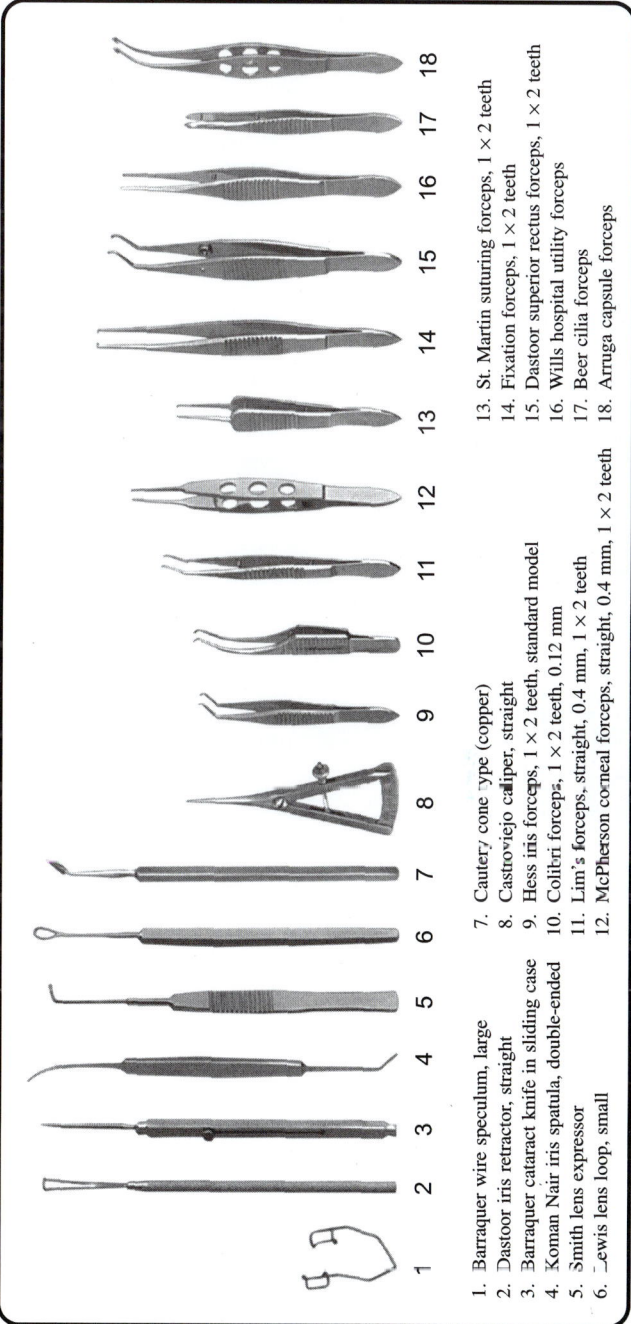

1. Barraquer wire speculum, large
2. Dastoor iris retractor, straight
3. Barraquer cataract knife in sliding case
4. Koman Nair iris spatula, double-ended
5. Smith lens expressor
6. Lewis lens loop, small
7. Cautery cone type (copper)
8. Castroviejo caliper, straight
9. Hess iris forceps, 1 × 2 teeth, standard model
10. Colibri forceps, 1 × 2 teeth, 0.12 mm
11. Lim's forceps, straight, 0.4 mm, 1 × 2 teeth
12. McPherson corneal forceps, straight, 0.4 mm, 1 × 2 teeth
13. St. Martin suturing forceps, 1 × 2 teeth
14. Fixation forceps, 1 × 2 teeth
15. Dastoor superior rectus forceps, 1 × 2 teeth
16. Wills hospital utility forceps
17. Beer cilia forceps
18. Arruga capsule forceps

Intracapsular Cataract Extraction Set (ICCE) (contd.)

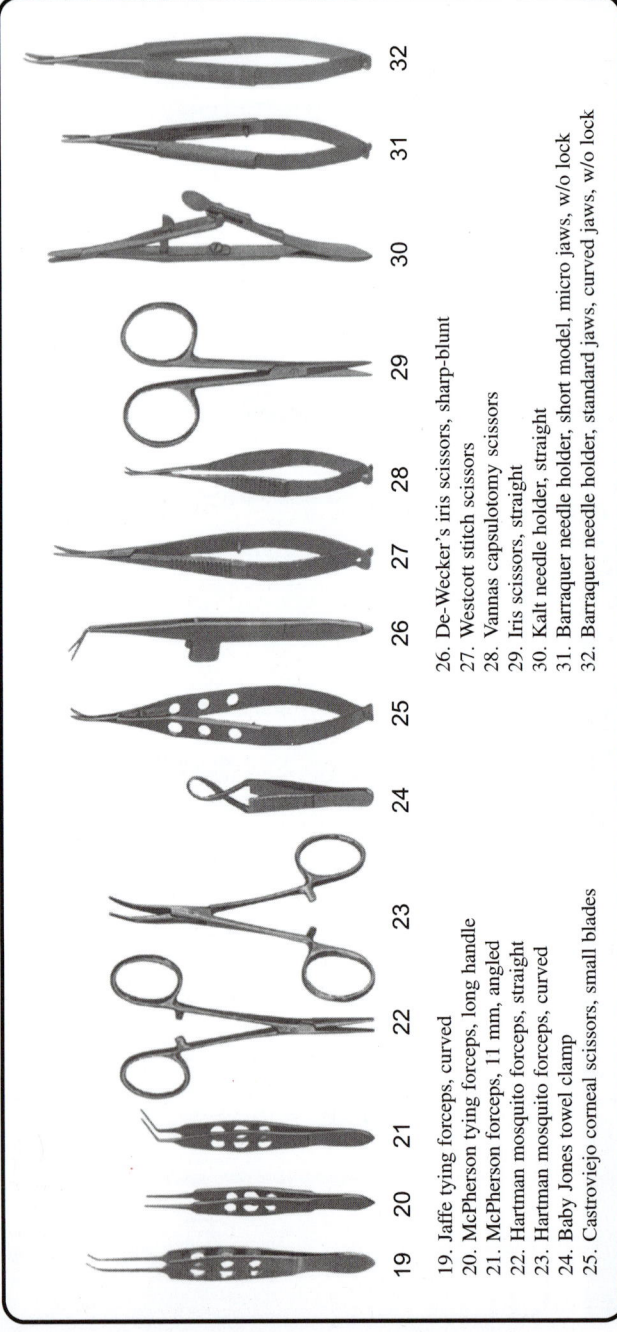

19. Jaffe tying forceps, curved
20. McPherson tying forceps, long handle
21. McPherson forceps, 11 mm, angled
22. Hartman mosquito forceps, straight
23. Hartman mosquito forceps, curved
24. Baby Jones towel clamp
25. Castroviejo corneal scissors, small blades
26. De-Wecker's iris scissors, sharp-blunt
27. Westcott stitch scissors
28. Vannas capsulotomy scissors
29. Iris scissors, straight
30. Kalt needle holder, straight
31. Barraquer needle holder, short model, micro jaws, w/o lock
32. Barraquer needle holder, standard jaws, curved jaws, w/o lock

Intracapsular Cataract Extraction Set (ICCE) (contd.)

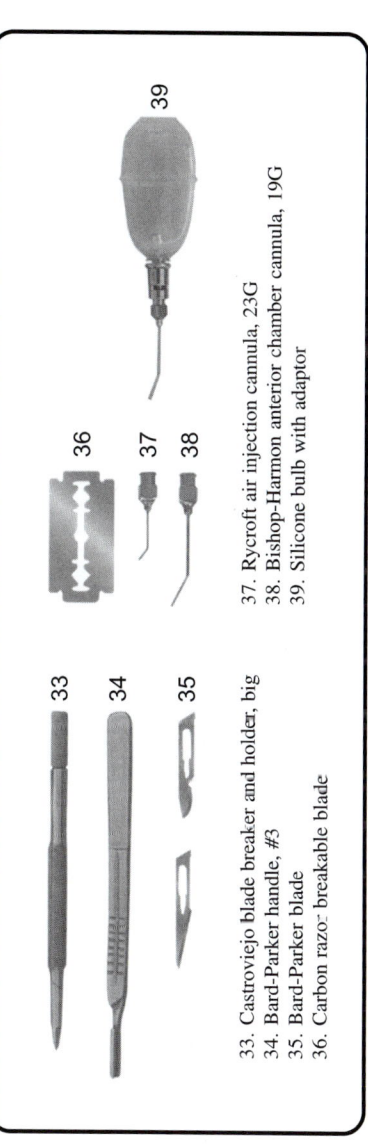

33. Castroviejo blade breaker and holder, big
34. Bard-Parker handle, #3
35. Bard-Parker blade
36. Carbon razor breakable blade
37. Rycroft air injection cannula, 23G
38. Bishop-Harmon anterior chamber cannula, 19G
39. Silicone bulb with adaptor

Extracapsular Cataract Extraction Set (ECCE)

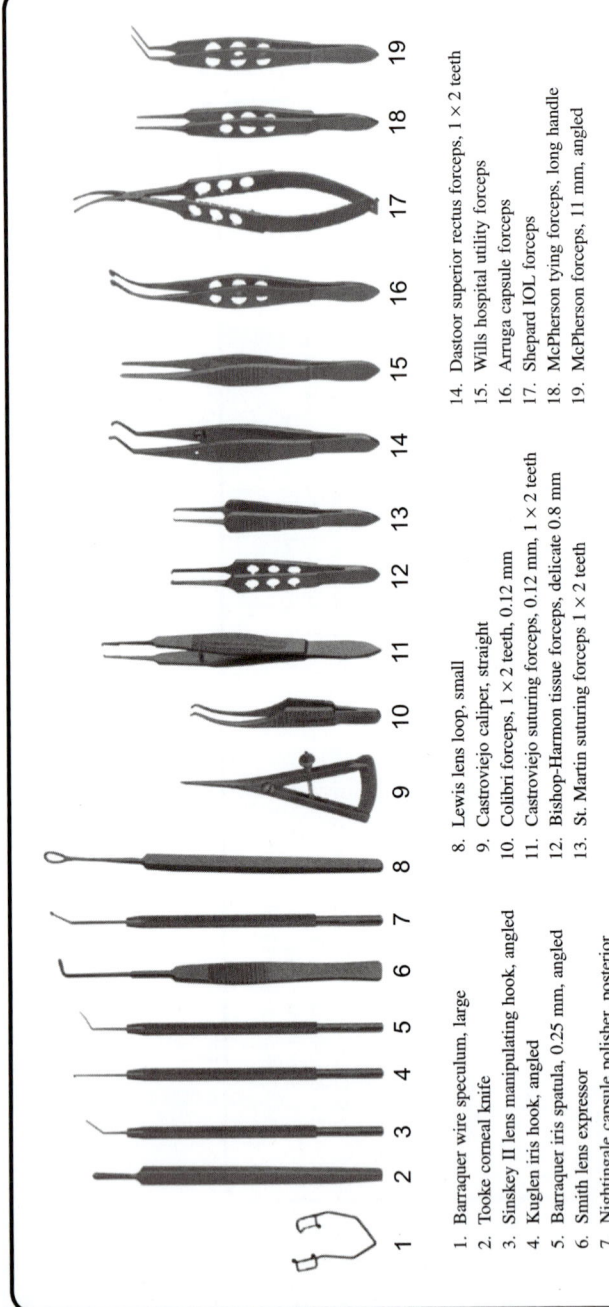

1. Barraquer wire speculum, large
2. Tooke corneal knife
3. Sinskey II lens manipulating hook, angled
4. Kuglen iris hook, angled
5. Barraquer iris spatula, 0.25 mm, angled
6. Smith lens expressor
7. Nightingale capsule polisher, posterior
8. Lewis lens loop, small
9. Castroviejo caliper, straight
10. Colibri forceps, 1 × 2 teeth, 0.12 mm
11. Castroviejo suturing forceps, 0.12 mm, 1 × 2 teeth
12. Bishop-Harmon tissue forceps, delicate 0.8 mm
13. St. Martin suturing forceps 1 × 2 teeth
14. Dastoor superior rectus forceps, 1 × 2 teeth
15. Wills hospital utility forceps
16. Arruga capsule forceps
17. Shepard IOL forceps
18. McPherson tying forceps, long handle
19. McPherson forceps, 11 mm, angled

Extracapsular Cataract Extraction Set (ECCE) (contd.)

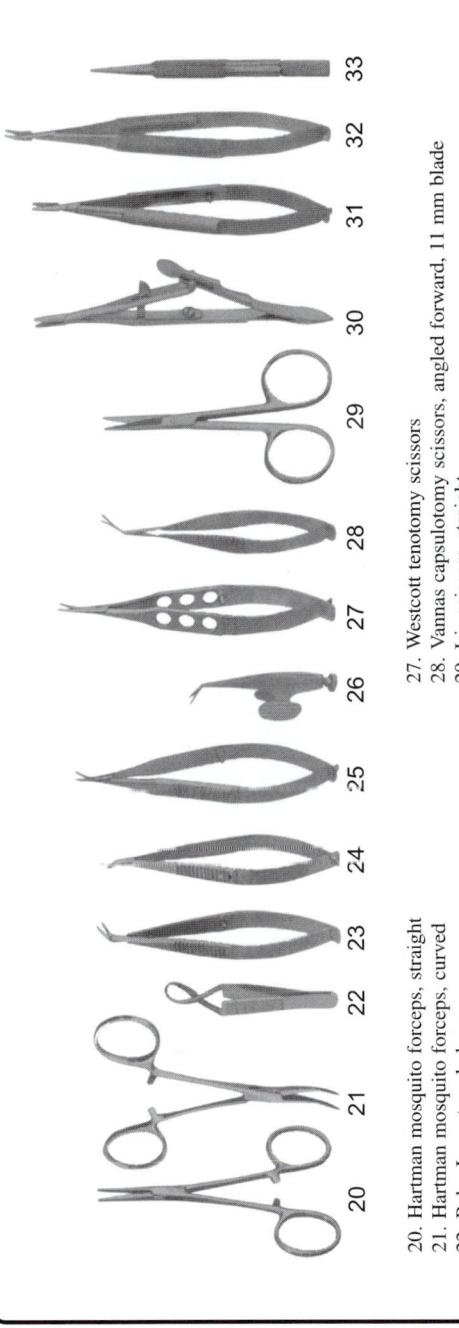

20. Hartman mosquito forceps, straight
21. Hartman mosquito forceps, curved
22. Baby Jones towel clamp
23. Castroviejo corneoscleral scissors, small blade, left
24. Castroviejo corneoscleral scissors, small blade, right
25. Micro iris scissors
26. Barraquer iris scissors
27. Westcott tenotomy scissors
28. Vannas capsulotomy scissors, angled forward, 11 mm blade
29. Iris scissors, straight
30. Kalt needle holder, straight
31. Barraquer needle holder, short model, micro jaws, curved, w/o lock
32. Barraquer needle holder, standard jaws, curved jaws, w/o lock
33. Swiss model blade breaker and holder, small

Extracapsular Cataract Extraction Set (ECCE) (contd.)

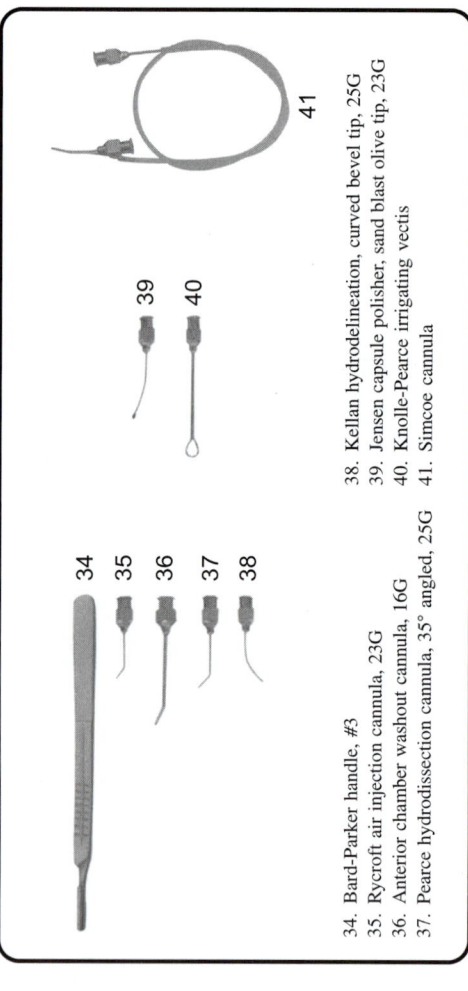

34. Bard-Parker handle, #3
35. Rycroft air injection cannula, 23G
36. Anterior chamber washout cannula, 16G
37. Pearce hydrodissection cannula, 35° angled, 25G
38. Kellan hydrodelineation, curved bevel tip, 25G
39. Jensen capsule polisher, sand blast olive tip, 23G
40. Knolle-Pearce irrigating vectis
41. Simcoe cannula

Small Incision Non-Phaco Set

Mini-Nucleus Technique (Blumenthal)

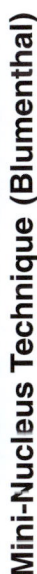

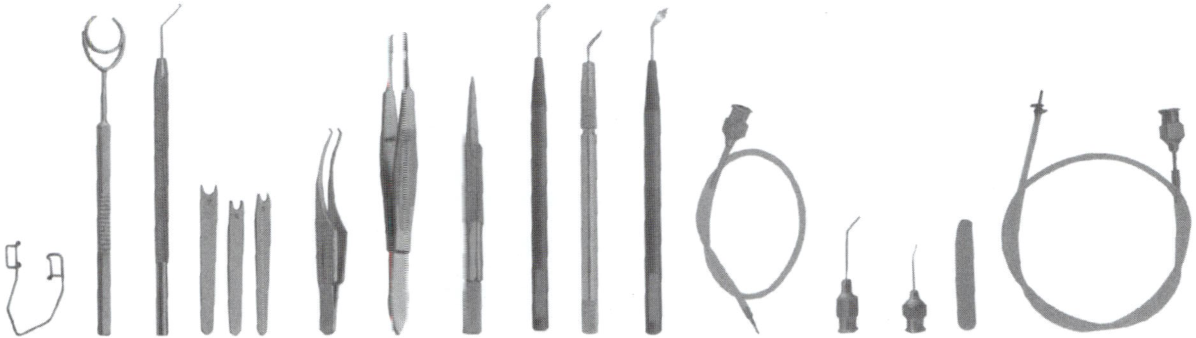

1. Barraquer wire speculum, large
2. Shepard fixation ring
3. Agarwal's phaco chopper, 1 mm fully cutting edge
4. Galand incision marker, size 3.0/3.5 mm
5. Colibri forceps, 1 × 2 teeth, 0.12 mm
6. Castrovejo suturing forceps, 0.12 mm, 1 × 2 teeth
7. Swiss model blade breaker and holder, small
8. Lance blade
9. Tunnel blade (crescent type)
10. Slit blade
11. Lewicky anterior chamber maintainer cannula
12. Blumenthal cannula, 25G
13. Blumenthal cannula, 27G
14. IOL glide 35 mm length × 5 mm wide
15. Infusion cannula, size 2.5 mm

Small Incision Non-Phaco Set (contd.)

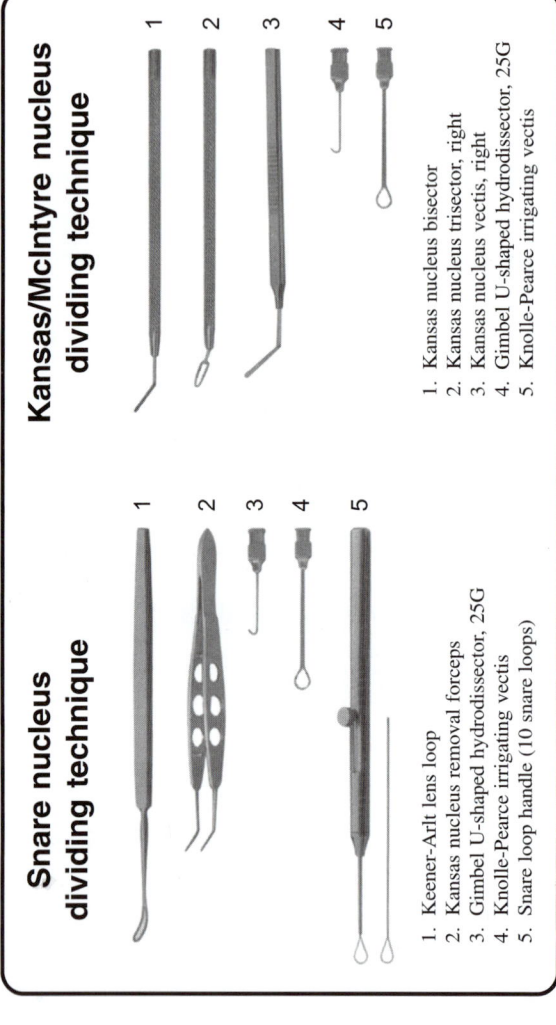

Snare nucleus dividing technique

1. Keener-Arlt lens loop
2. Kansas nucleus removal forceps
3. Gimbel U-shaped hydrodissector, 25G
4. Knolle-Pearce irrigating vectis
5. Snare loop handle (10 snare loops)

Kansas/McIntyre nucleus dividing technique

1. Kansas nucleus bisector
2. Kansas nucleus trisector, right
3. Kansas nucleus vectis, right
4. Gimbel U-shaped hydrodissector, 25G
5. Knolle-Pearce irrigating vectis

ECCE-Phaco Emulsification Set

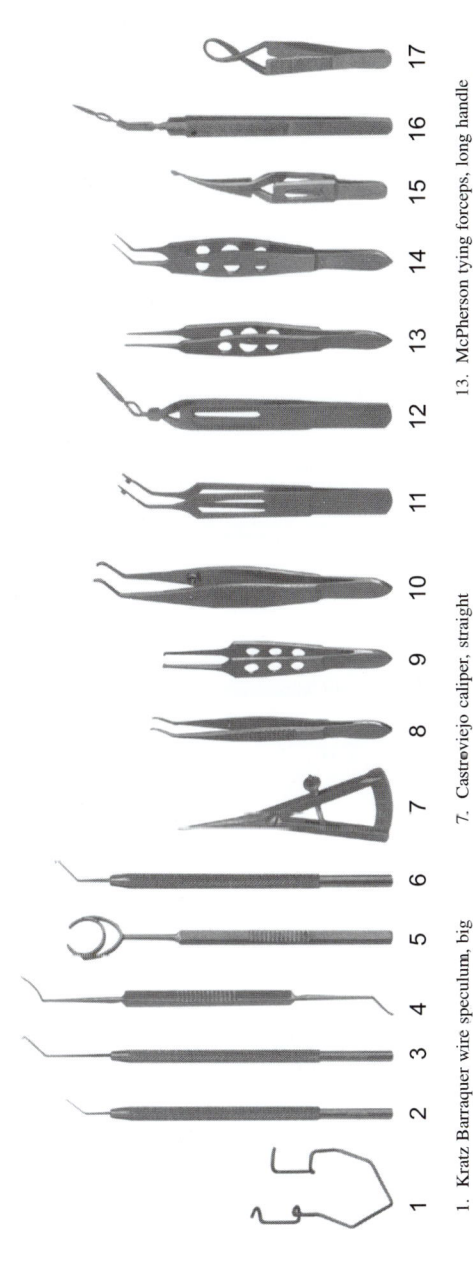

1. Kratz Barraquer wire speculum, big
2. Sinskey II lens manipulating hook, angled
3. Akahoshi nucleus sustainer
4. Castroviejo cyclodialysis spatula, 0.50 mm wide
5. Shepard fixation ring
6. Agarwal's phaco chopper, 1 mm fully cutting edge
7. Castroviejo caliper, straight
8. Lim's corneoscleral forceps, 0.12 mm, 1 × 2 teeth
9. Bishop-Harmon tissue forceps, delicate, 0.8 mm
10. Dastoor superior rectus forceps, 1 × 2 teeth
11. Appa-amy lens folder
12. Appa-amy lens inserting forceps
13. McPherson tying forceps, long handle
14. Utrata capsulorhexis forceps, flat handle
15. Dodick nucleus cracker
16. Akahoshi prechop forceps, curved shanks
17. Baby Jones towel clamp

ECCE-Phaco Emulsification Set (contd.)

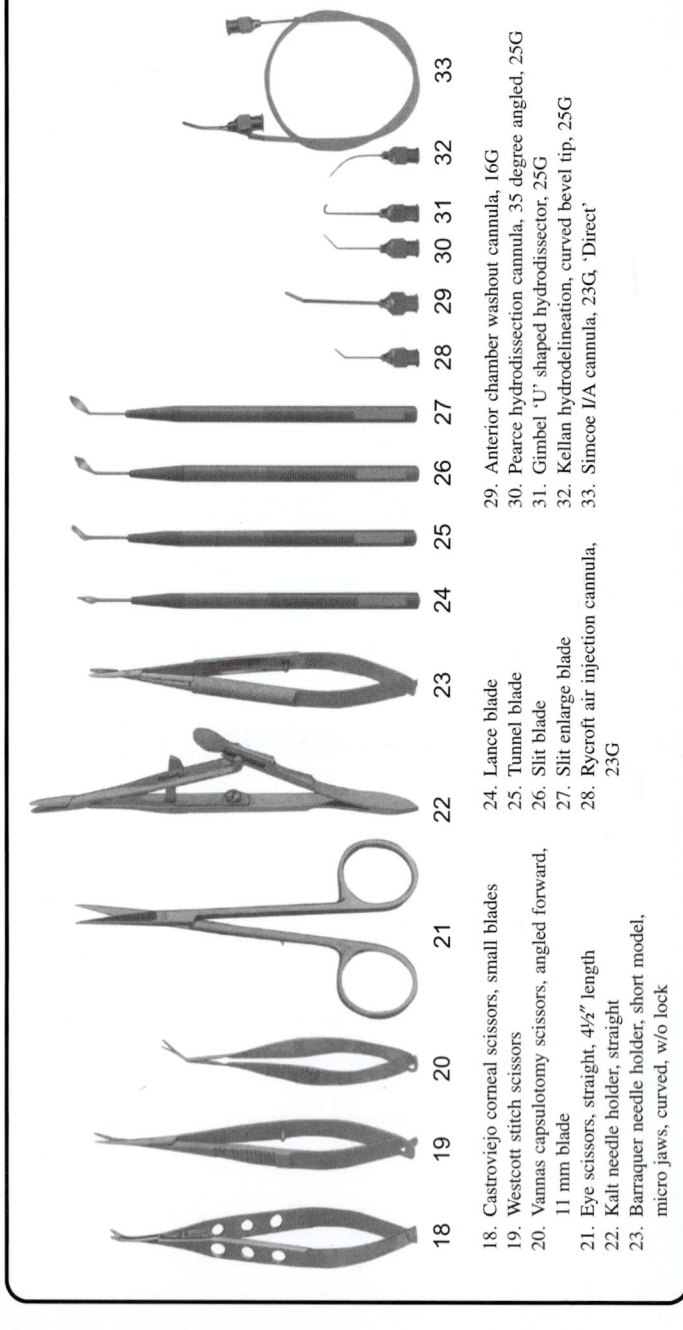

18. Castroviejo corneal scissors, small blades
19. Westcott stitch scissors
20. Vannas capsulotomy scissors, angled forward, 11 mm blade
21. Eye scissors, straight, 4½" length
22. Kalt needle holder, straight
23. Barraquer needle holder, short model, micro jaws, curved, w/o lock

24. Lance blade
25. Tunnel blade
26. Slit blade
27. Slit enlarge blade
28. Rycroft air injection cannula, 23G

29. Anterior chamber washout cannula, 16G
30. Pearce hydrodissection cannula, 35 degree angled, 25G
31. Gimbel 'U' shaped hydrodissector, 25G
32. Kellan hydrodelineation, curved bevel tip, 25G
33. Simcoe I/A cannula, 23G, 'Direct'

Specific Instruments Set for Phaconit

MICS (Micro Incision Cataract Surgery)

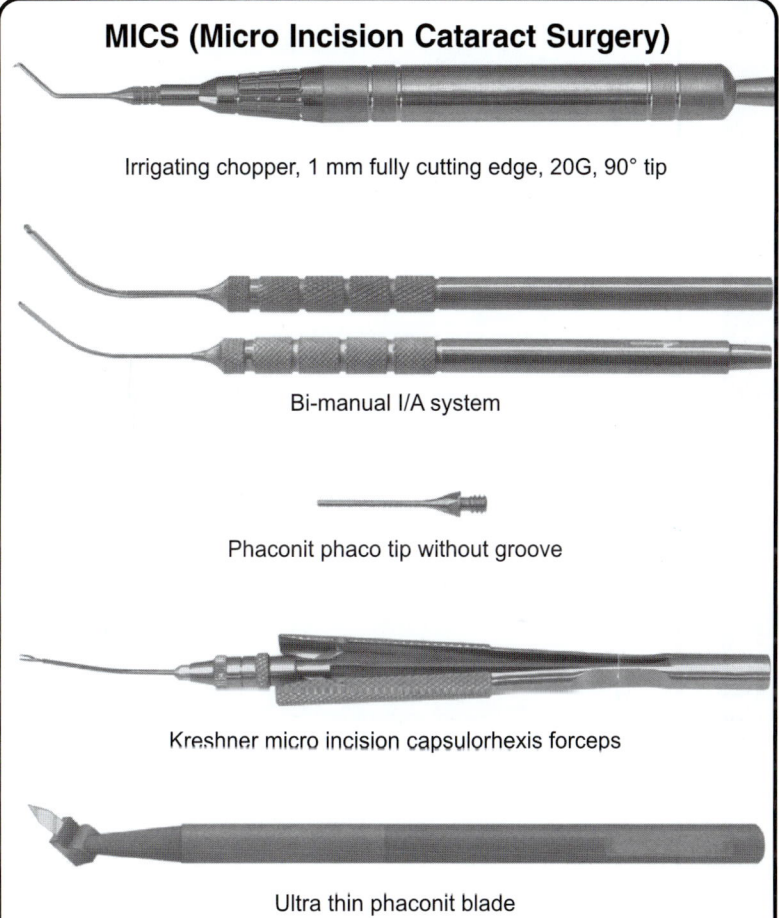

Irrigating chopper, 1 mm fully cutting edge, 20G, 90° tip

Bi-manual I/A system

Phaconit phaco tip without groove

Kreshner micro incision capsulorhexis forceps

Ultra thin phaconit blade

Specific Instruments Set for IOL

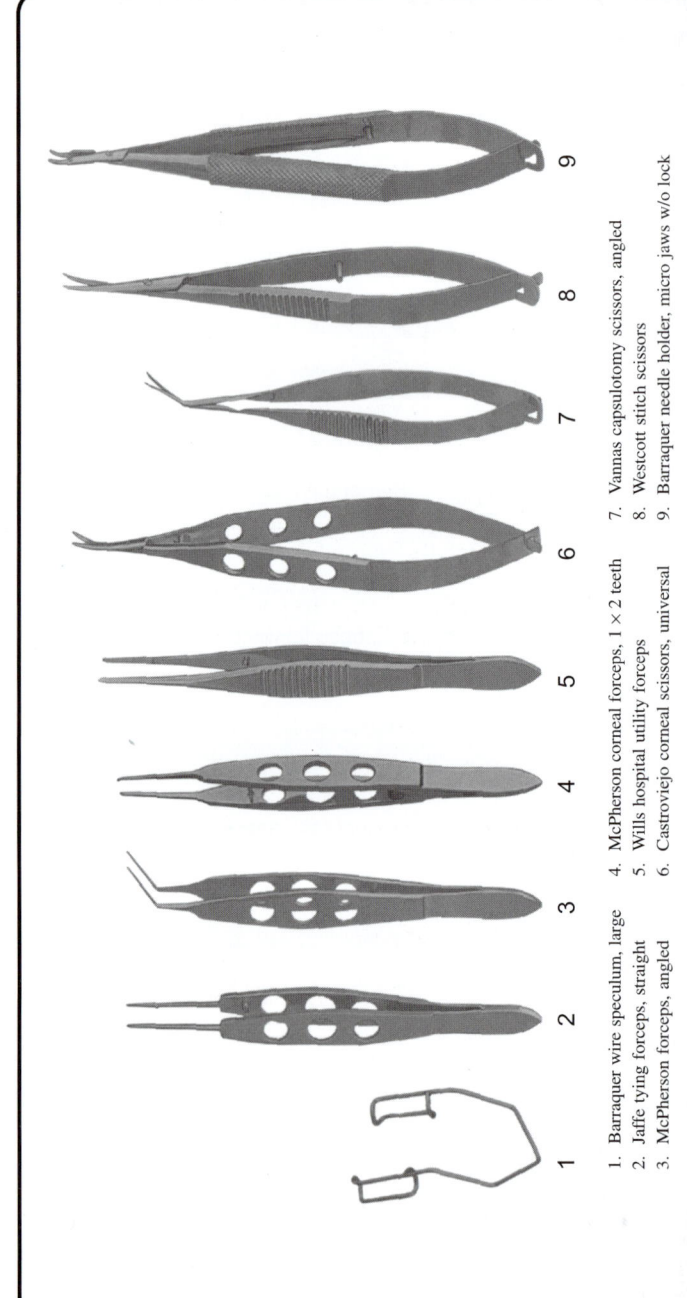

1. Barraquer wire speculum, large
2. Jaffe tying forceps, straight
3. McPherson forceps, angled
4. McPherson corneal forceps, 1 × 2 teeth
5. Wills hospital utility forceps
6. Castroviejo corneal scissors, universal
7. Vannas capsulotomy scissors, angled
8. Westcott stitch scissors
9. Barraquer needle holder, micro jaws w/o lock

Specific Instruments Set for IOL (contd.)

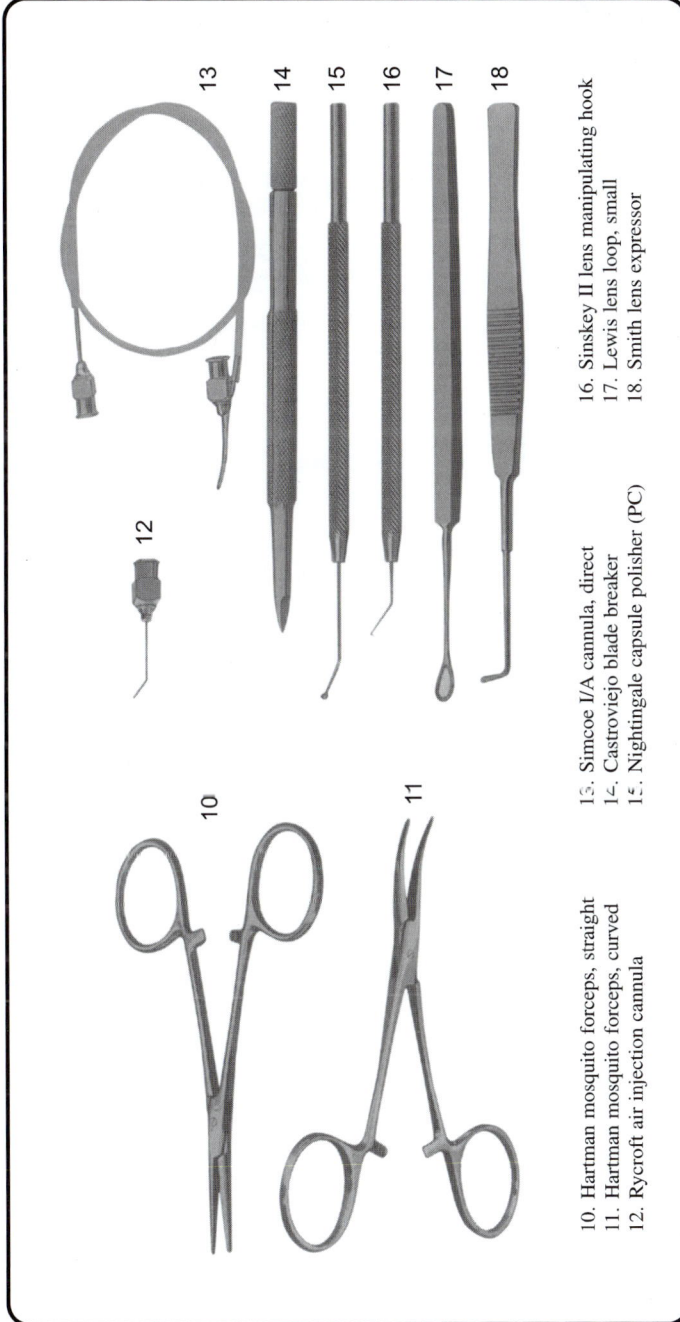

10. Hartman mosquito forceps, straight
11. Hartman mosquito forceps, curved
12. Rycroft air injection cannula

13. Simcoe I/A cannula, direct
14. Castroviejo blade breaker
15. Nightingale capsule polisher (PC)

16. Sinskey II lens manipulating hook
17. Lewis lens loop, small
18. Smith lens expressor

GLAUCOMA

Glaucoma Surgery Set

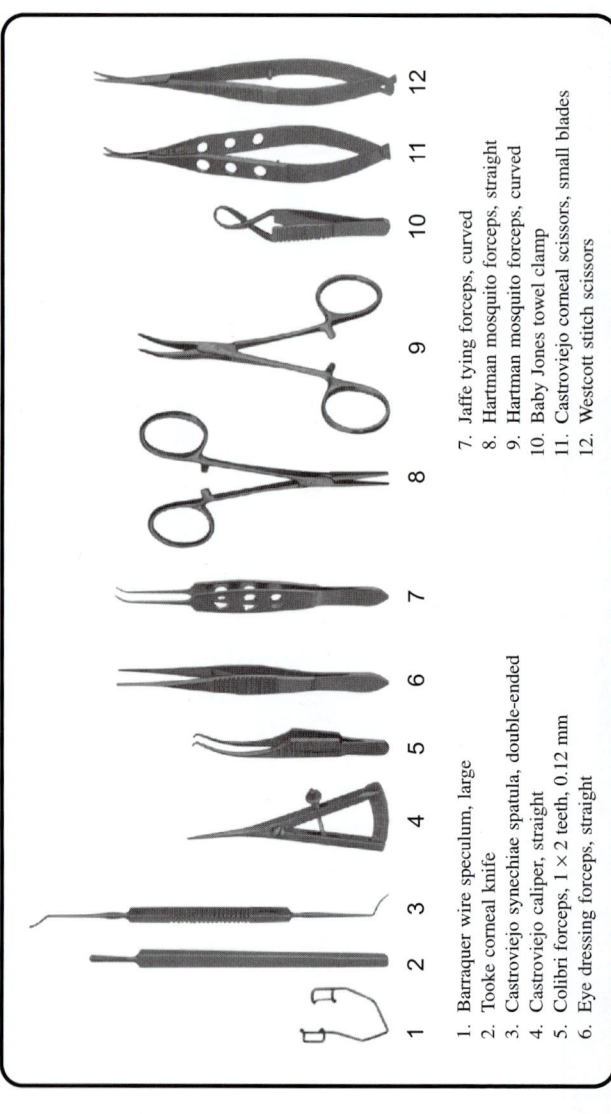

1. Barraquer wire speculum, large
2. Tooke corneal knife
3. Castroviejo synechiae spatula, double-ended
4. Castroviejo caliper, straight
5. Colibri forceps, 1 × 2 teeth, 0.12 mm
6. Eye dressing forceps, straight
7. Jaffe tying forceps, curved
8. Hartman mosquito forceps, straight
9. Hartman mosquito forceps, curved
10. Baby Jones towel clamp
11. Castroviejo corneal scissors, small blades
12. Westcott stitch scissors

Glaucoma Surgery Set (contd.)

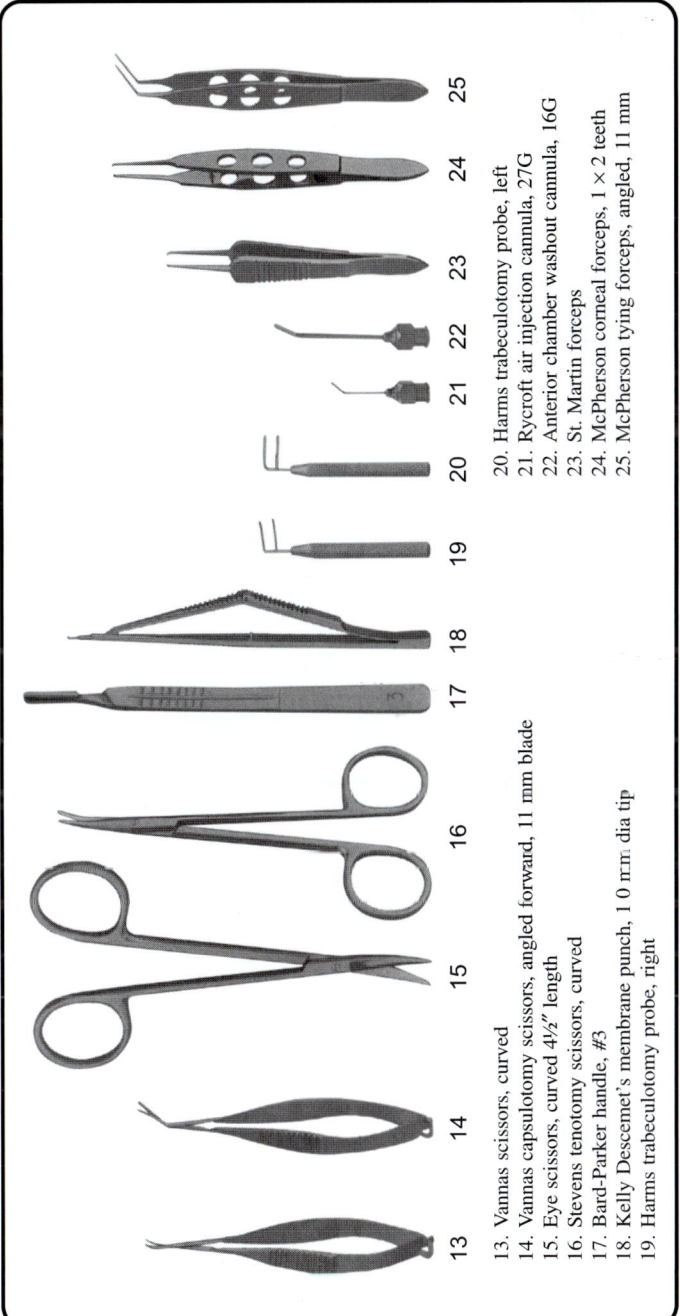

13. Vannas scissors, curved
14. Vannas capsulotomy scissors, angled forward, 11 mm blade
15. Eye scissors, curved 4½" length
16. Stevens tenotomy scissors, curved
17. Bard-Parker handle, #3
18. Kelly Descemet's membrane punch, 1 0 mm dia tip
19. Harms trabeculotomy probe, right
20. Harms trabeculotomy probe, left
21. Rycroft air injection cannula, 27G
22. Anterior chamber washout cannula, 16G
23. St. Martin forceps
24. McPherson corneal forceps, 1 × 2 teeth
25. McPherson tying forceps, angled, 11 mm

CORNEA

Corneal Transplant Set

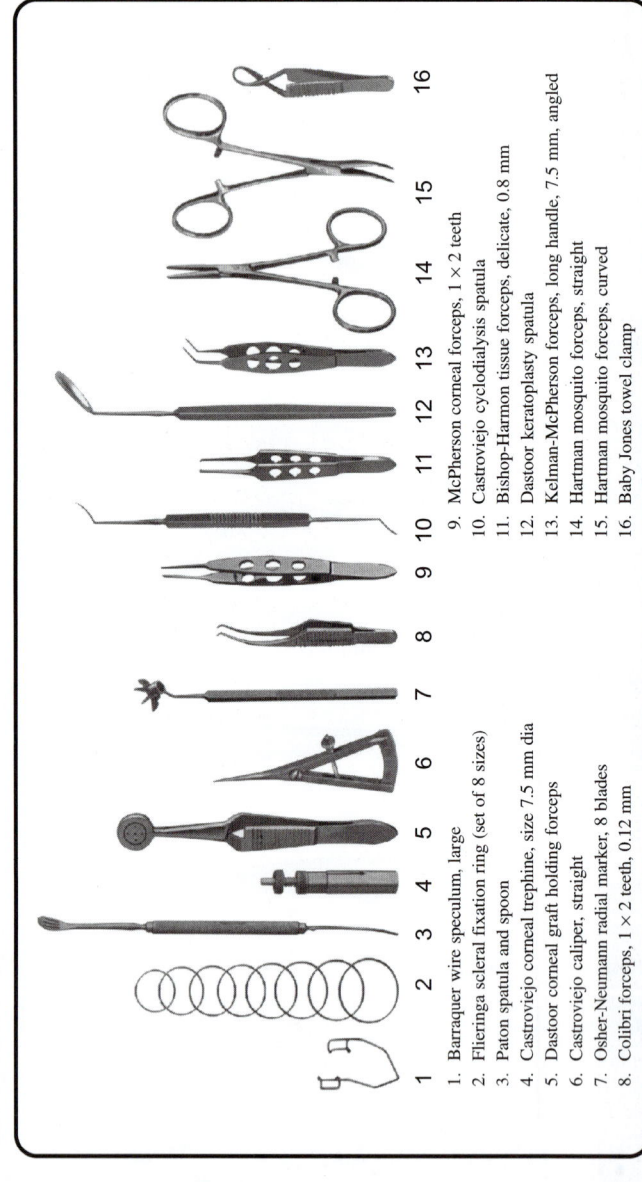

1. Barraquer wire speculum, large
2. Flieringa scleral fixation ring (set of 8 sizes)
3. Paton spatula and spoon
4. Castroviejo corneal trephine, size 7.5 mm dia
5. Dastoor corneal graft holding forceps
6. Castroviejo caliper, straight
7. Osher-Neumann radial marker, 8 blades
8. Colibri forceps, 1 × 2 teeth, 0.12 mm
9. McPherson corneal forceps, 1 × 2 teeth
10. Castroviejo cyclodialysis spatula
11. Bishop-Harmon tissue forceps, delicate, 0.8 mm
12. Dastoor keratoplasty spatula
13. Kelman-McPherson forceps, long handle, 7.5 mm, angled
14. Hartman mosquito forceps, straight
15. Hartman mosquito forceps, curved
16. Baby Jones towel clamp

Corneal Transplant Set (contd.)

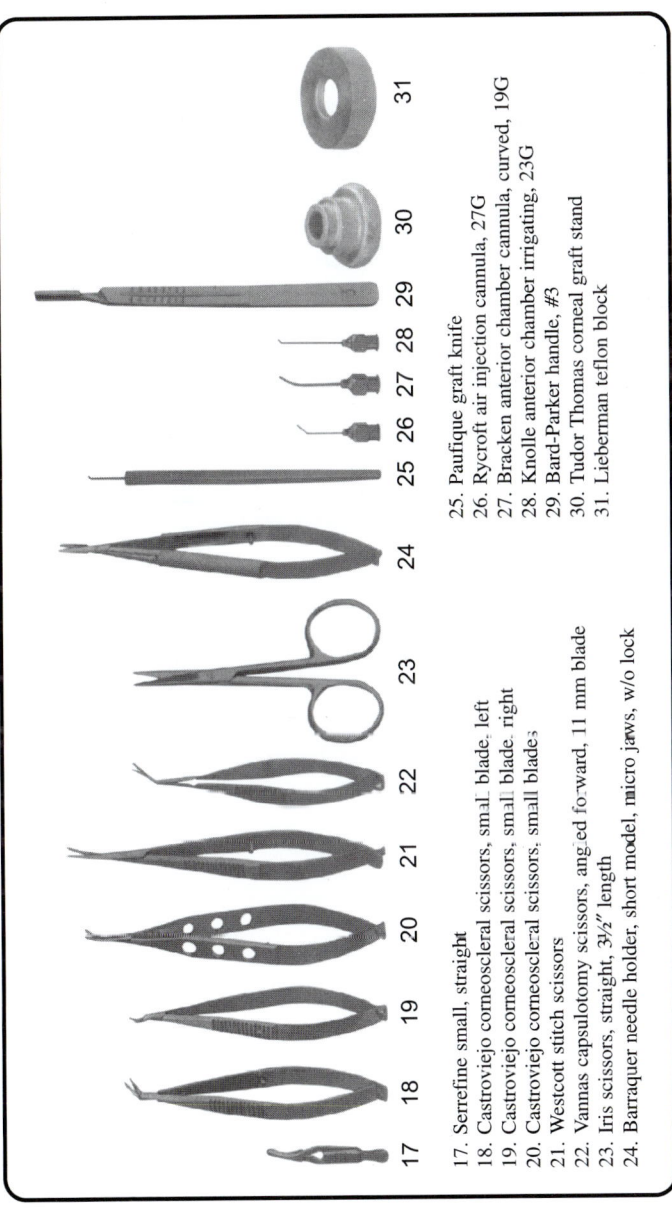

17. Serrefine small, straight
18. Castroviejo corneoscleral scissors, small blade, left
19. Castroviejo corneoscleral scissors, small blade, right
20. Castroviejo corneoscleral scissors, small blade,
21. Westcott stitch scissors
22. Vannas capsulotomy scissors, angled forward, 11 mm blade
23. Iris scissors, straight, 3½" length
24. Barraquer needle holder, short model, micro jaws, w/o lock

25. Paufique graft knife
26. Rycroft air injection cannula, 27G
27. Bracken anterior chamber cannula, curved, 19G
28. Knolle anterior chamber irrigating, 23G
29. Bard-Parker handle, #3
30. Tudor Thomas corneal graft stand
31. Lieberman teflon block

Specific Instruments Set for DSAEK

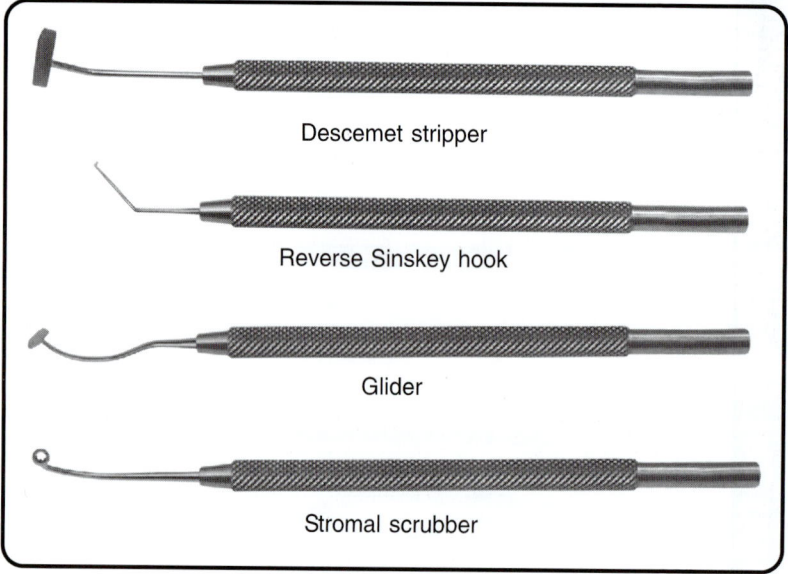

Descemet stripper

Reverse Sinskey hook

Glider

Stromal scrubber

Specific Instruments Set for Radial Keratotomy

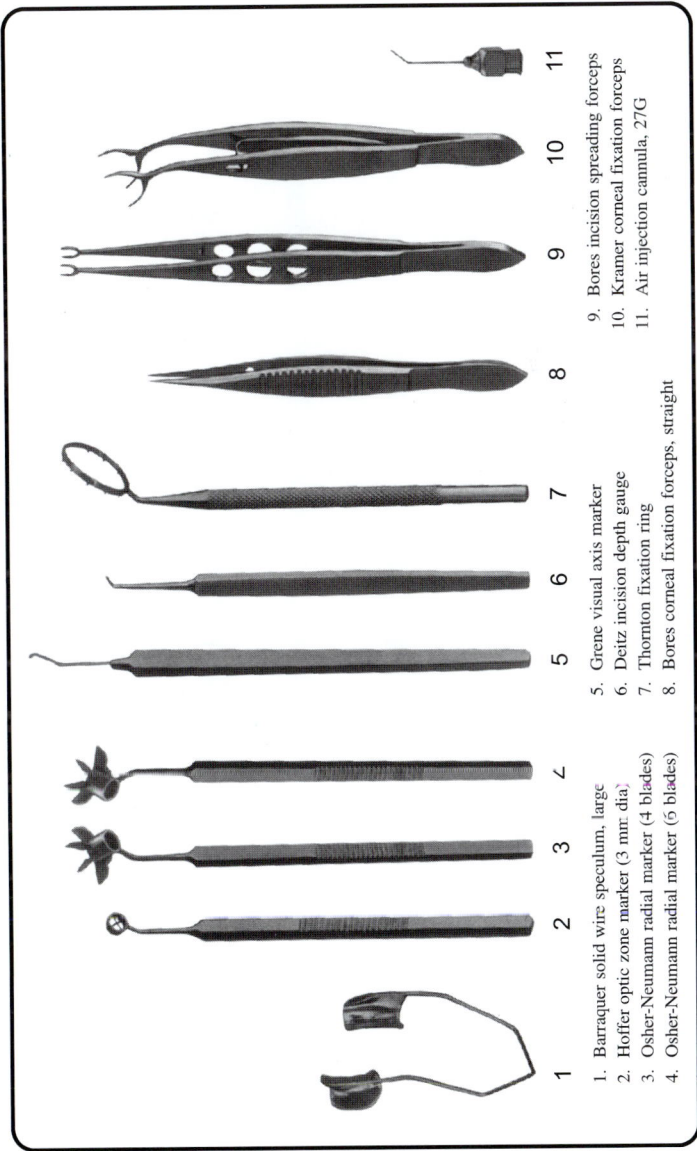

1. Barraquer solid wire speculum, large
2. Hoffer optic zone marker (3 mm dia.)
3. Osher-Neumann radial marker (4 blades)
4. Osher-Neumann radial marker (5 blades)
5. Grene visual axis marker
6. Deitz incision depth gauge
7. Thornton fixation ring
8. Bores corneal fixation forceps, straight
9. Bores incision spreading forceps
10. Kramer corneal fixation forceps
11. Air injection cannula, 27G

Specific Instruments Set for LASIK

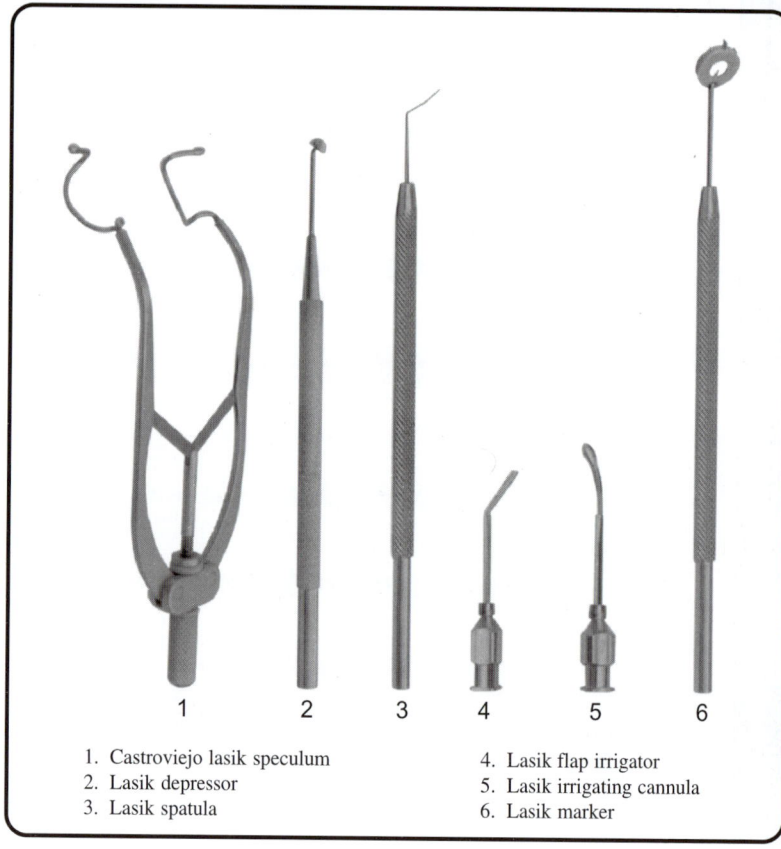

1. Castroviejo lasik speculum
2. Lasik depressor
3. Lasik spatula
4. Lasik flap irrigator
5. Lasik irrigating cannula
6. Lasik marker

Pterygium Surgery Set

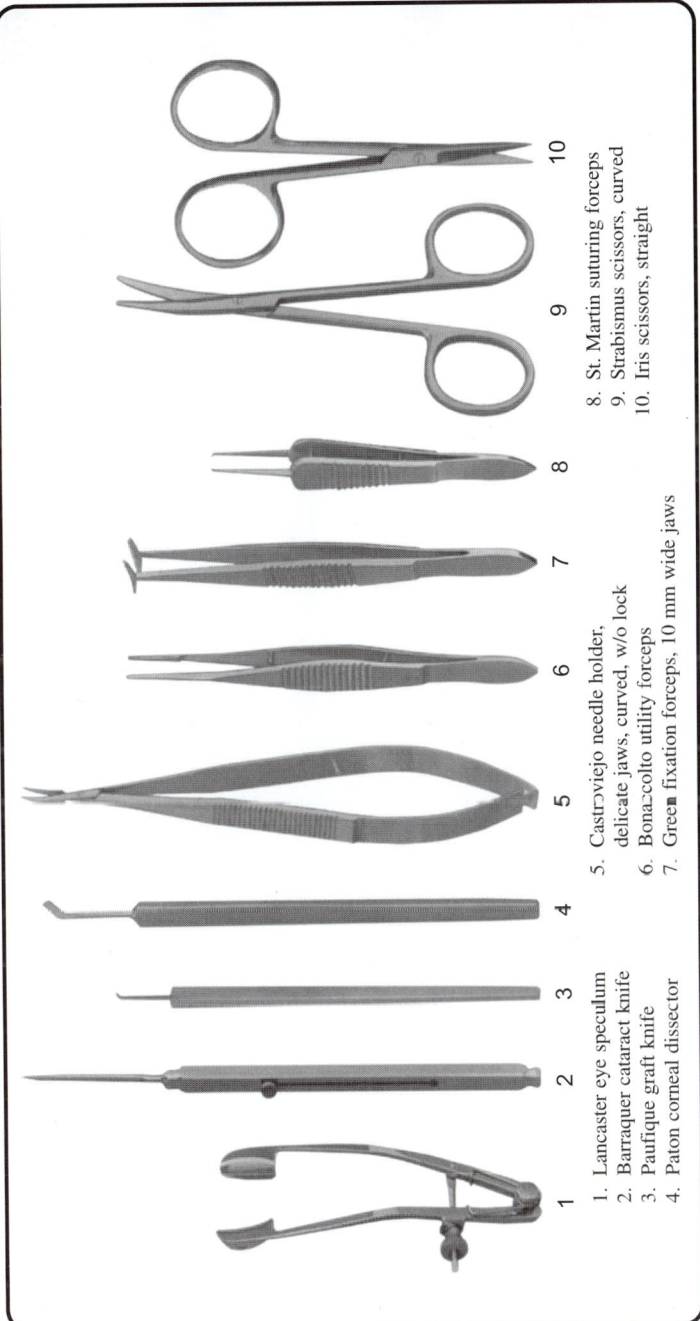

1. Lancaster eye speculum
2. Barraquer cataract knife
3. Paufique graft knife
4. Paton corneal dissector
5. Castroviejo needle holder, delicate jaws, curved, w/o lock
6. Bonaccolto utility forceps
7. Green fixation forceps, 10 mm wide jaws
8. St. Martin suturing forceps
9. Strabismus scissors, curved
10. Iris scissors, straight

Foreign Body Removal Set

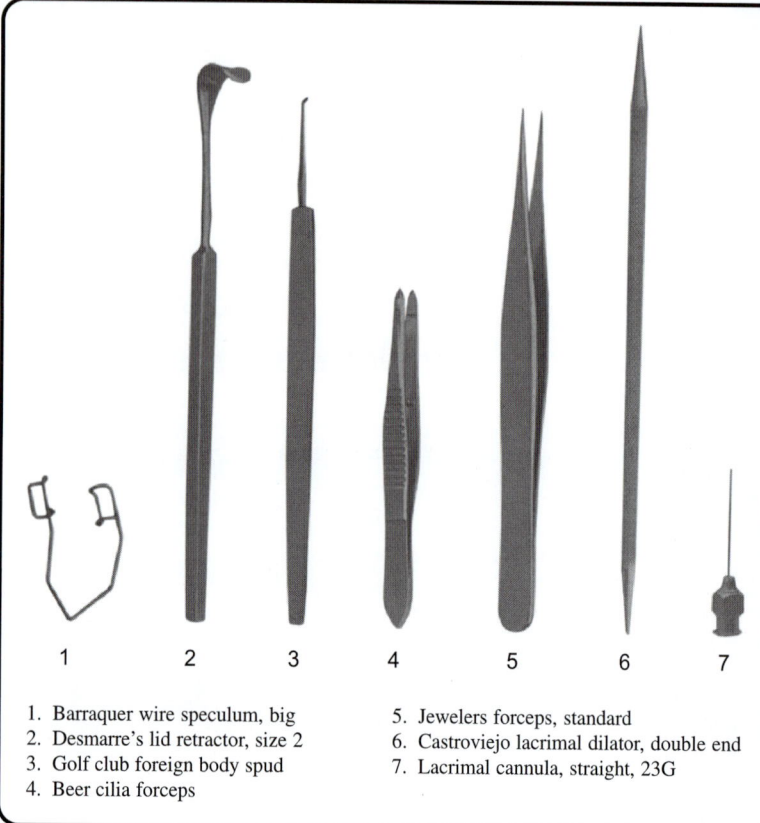

1. Barraquer wire speculum, big
2. Desmarre's lid retractor, size 2
3. Golf club foreign body spud
4. Beer cilia forceps
5. Jewelers forceps, standard
6. Castroviejo lacrimal dilator, double end
7. Lacrimal cannula, straight, 23G

RETINA

Retinal Surgery Set

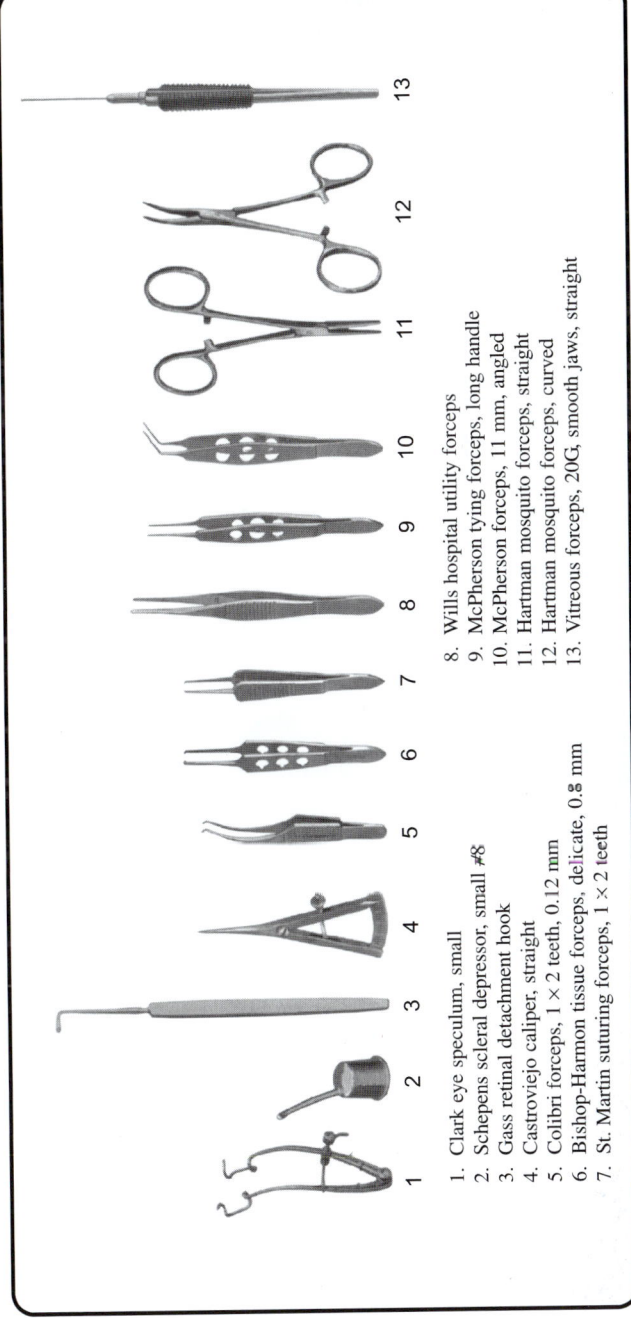

1. Clark eye speculum, small
2. Schepens scleral depressor, small #8
3. Gass retinal detachment hook
4. Castroviejo caliper, straight
5. Colibri forceps, 1 × 2 teeth, 0.12 mm
6. Bishop-Harmon tissue forceps, delicate, 0.8 mm
7. St. Martin suturing forceps, 1 × 2 teeth
8. Wills hospital utility forceps
9. McPherson tying forceps, long handle
10. McPherson forceps, 11 mm, angled
11. Hartman mosquito forceps, straight
12. Hartman mosquito forceps, curved
13. Vitreous forceps, 20G, smooth jaws, straight

Retinal Surgery Set (contd.)

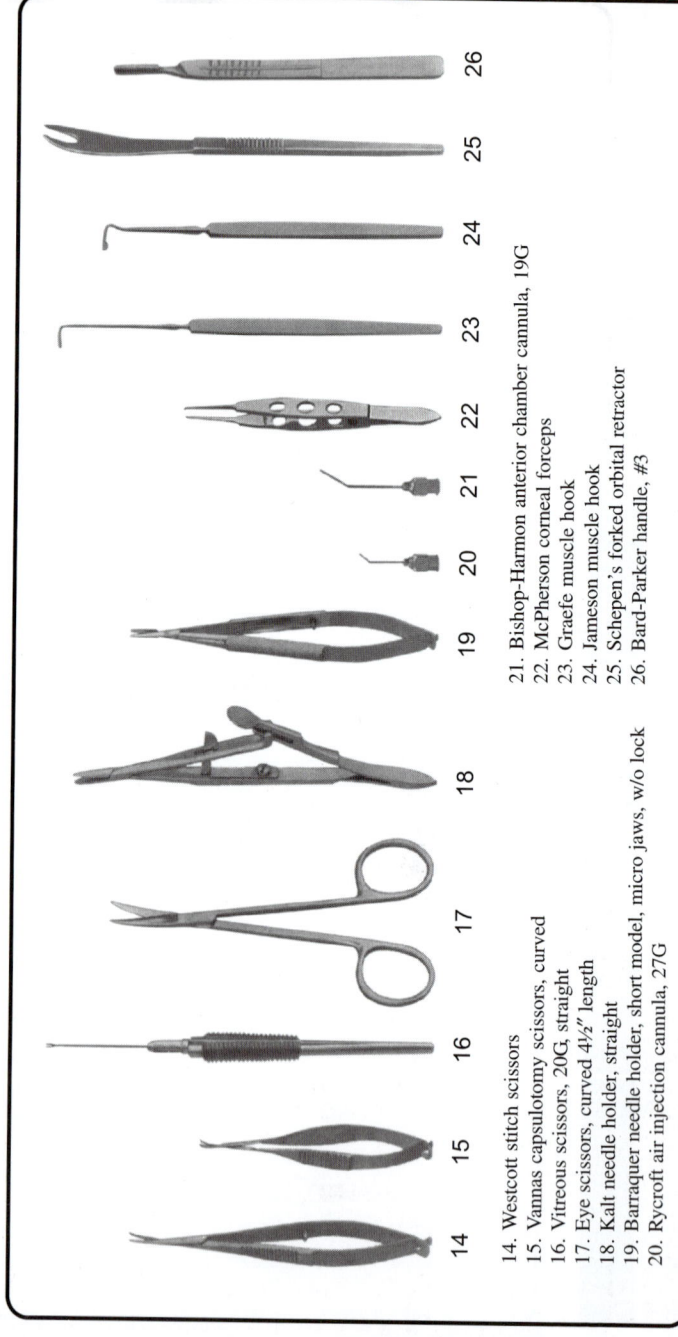

14. Westcott stitch scissors
15. Vannas capsulotomy scissors, curved
16. Vitreous scissors, 20G, straight
17. Eye scissors, curved 4½" length
18. Kalt needle holder, straight
19. Barraquer needle holder, short model, micro jaws, w/o lock
20. Rycroft air injection cannula, 27G
21. Bishop-Harmon anterior chamber cannula, 19G
22. McPherson corneal forceps
23. Graefe muscle hook
24. Jameson muscle hook
25. Schepen's forked orbital retractor
26. Bard-Parker handle, #3

Vitreo-Retinal Surgery Set

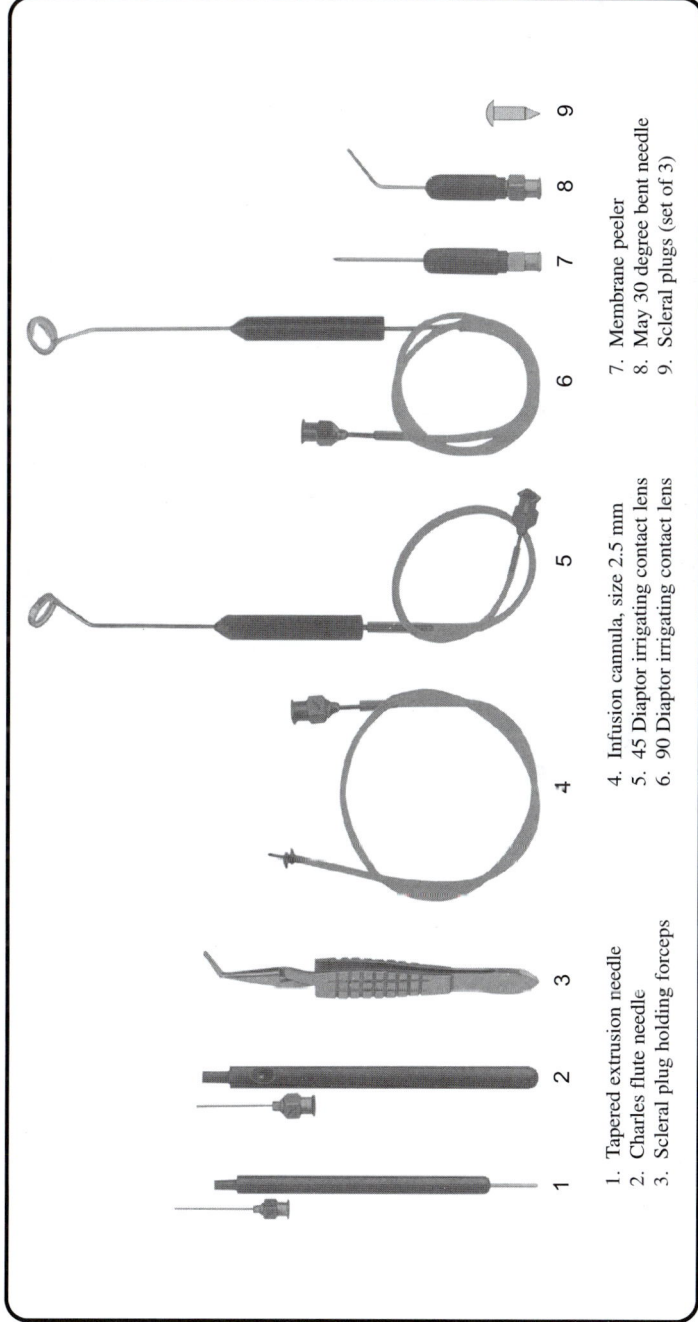

1. Tapered extrusion needle
2. Charles flute needle
3. Scleral plug holding forceps
4. Infusion cannula, size 2.5 mm
5. 45 Diaptor irrigating contact lens
6. 90 Diaptor irrigating contact lens
7. Membrane peeler
8. May 30 degree bent needle
9. Scleral plugs (set of 3)

LID AND ADNEXA

Lid Surgery Set

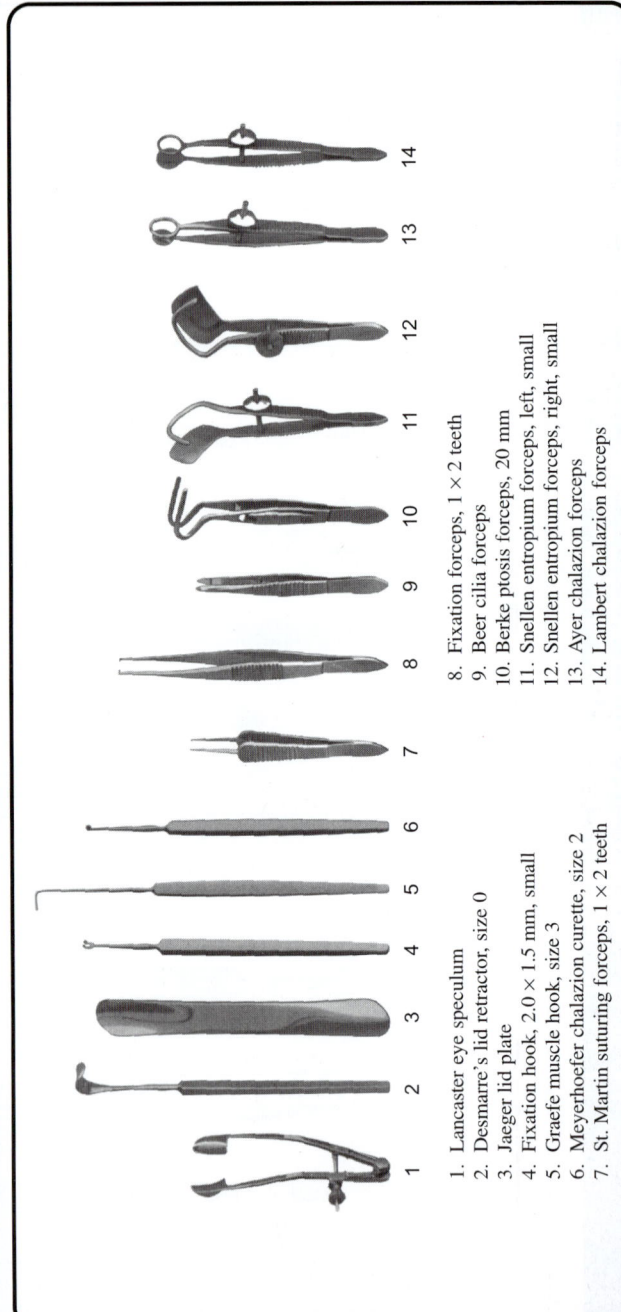

1. Lancaster eye speculum
2. Desmarre's lid retractor, size 0
3. Jaeger lid plate
4. Fixation hook, 2.0 × 1.5 mm, small
5. Graefe muscle hook, size 3
6. Meyerhoefer chalazion curette, size 2
7. St. Martin suturing forceps, 1 × 2 teeth
8. Fixation forceps, 1 × 2 teeth
9. Beer cilia forceps
10. Berke ptosis forceps, 20 mm
11. Snellen entropium forceps, left, small
12. Snellen entropium forceps, right, small
13. Ayer chalazion forceps
14. Lambert chalazion forceps

Lid Surgery Set (contd.)

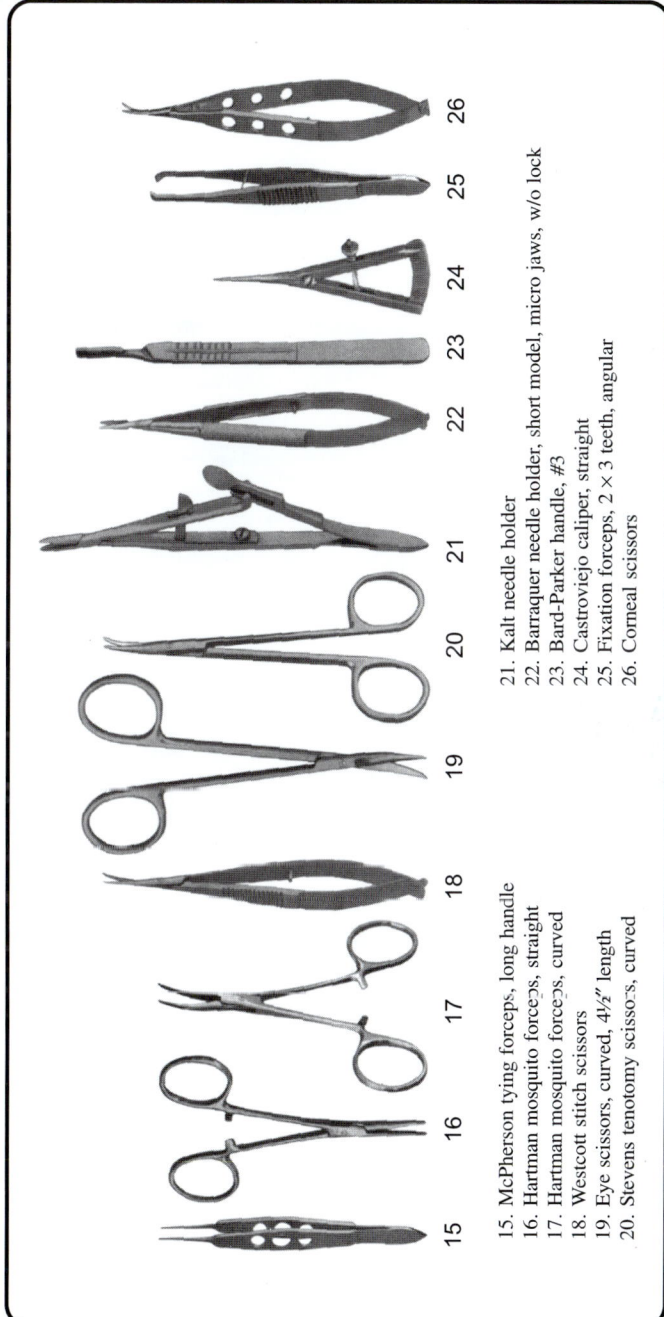

15. McPherson tying forceps, long handle
16. Hartman mosquito forceps, straight
17. Hartman mosquito forceps, curved
18. Westcott stitch scissors
19. Eye scissors, curved, 4½″ length
20. Stevens tenotomy scissors, curved

21. Kalt needle holder
22. Barraquer needle holder, short model, micro jaws, w/o lock
23. Bard-Parker handle, #3
24. Castroviejo caliper, straight
25. Fixation forceps, 2 × 3 teeth, angular
26. Corneal scissors

Chalazion Surgery Set

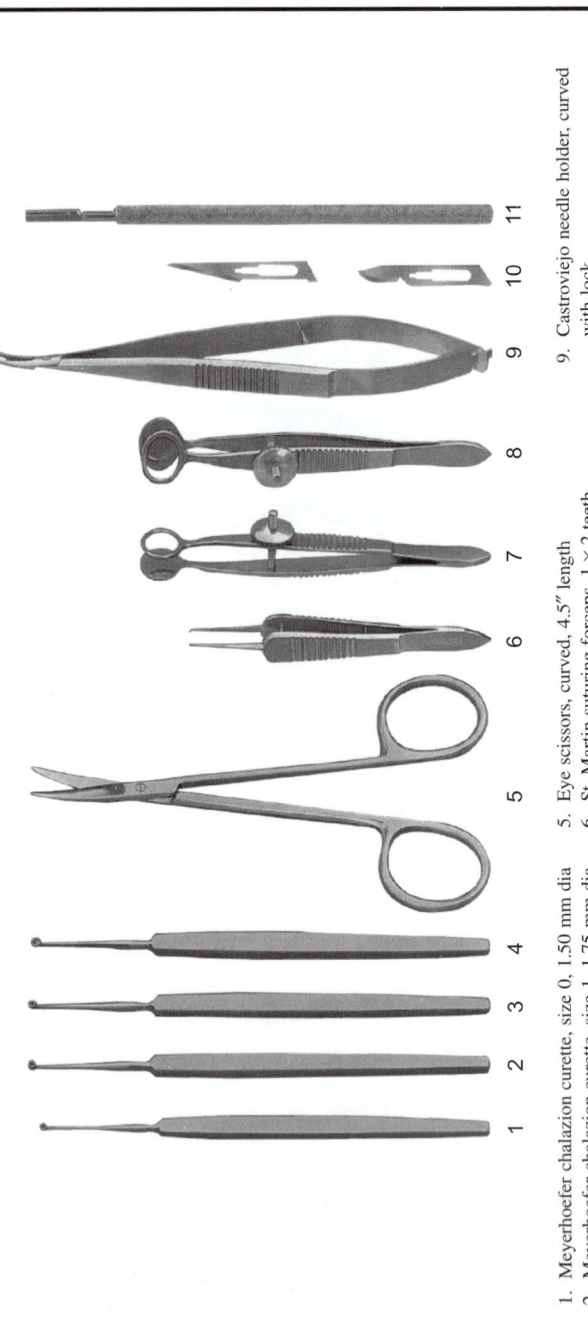

1. Meyerhoefer chalazion curette, size 0, 1.50 mm dia
2. Meyerhoefer chalazion curette, size 1, 1.75 mm dia
3. Meyerhoefer chalazion curette, size 2, 2.25 mm dia
4. Meyerhoefer chalazion curette, size 3, 3.0 mm dia
5. Eye scissors, curved, 4.5" length
6. St. Martin suturing forceps, 1 × 2 teeth
7. Hunt chalazion forceps, 12 mm dia
8. Desmarre's chalazion forceps, 13 mm/20 mm dia
9. Castroviejo needle holder, curved with lock
10. Bard-Parker blade, #11, #15
11. Bard-Parker handle, #3, round handle

Lacrimal Sac Surgery Set

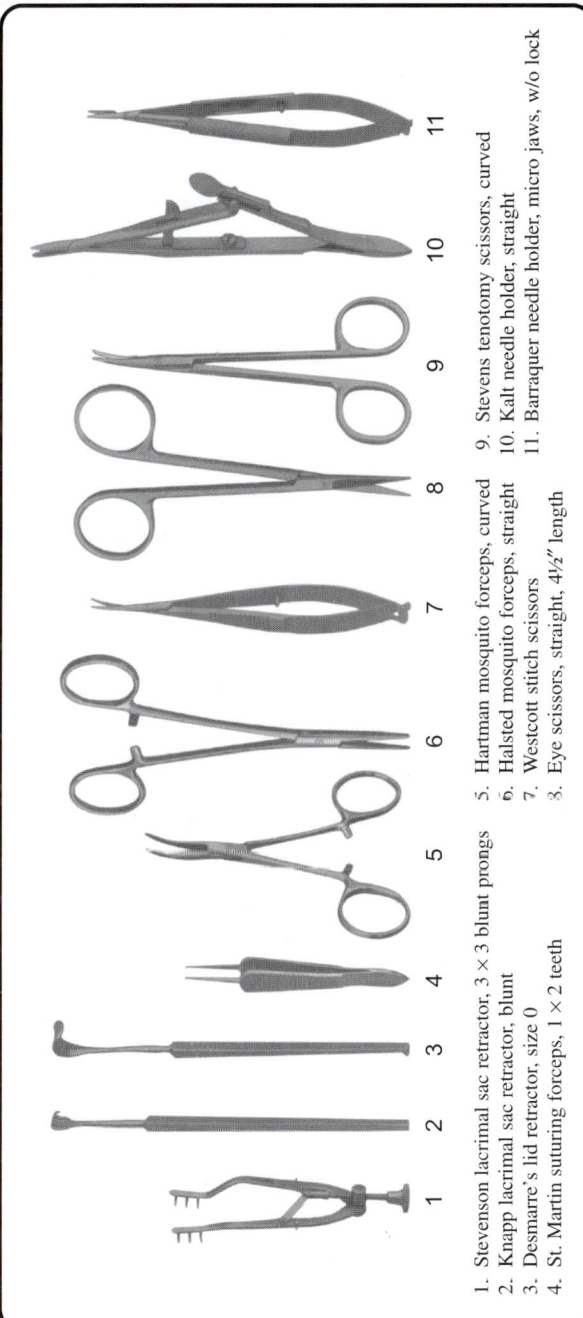

1. Stevenson lacrimal sac retractor, 3 × 3 blunt prongs
2. Knapp lacrimal sac retractor, blunt
3. Desmarre's lid retractor, size 0
4. St. Martin suturing forceps, 1 × 2 teeth
5. Hartman mosquito forceps, curved
6. Halsted mosquito forceps, straight
7. Westcott stitch scissors
8. Eye scissors, straight, 4½″ length
9. Stevens tenotomy scissors, curved
10. Kalt needle holder, straight
11. Barraquer needle holder, micro jaws, w/o lock

Lacrimal Sac Surgery Set (contd.)

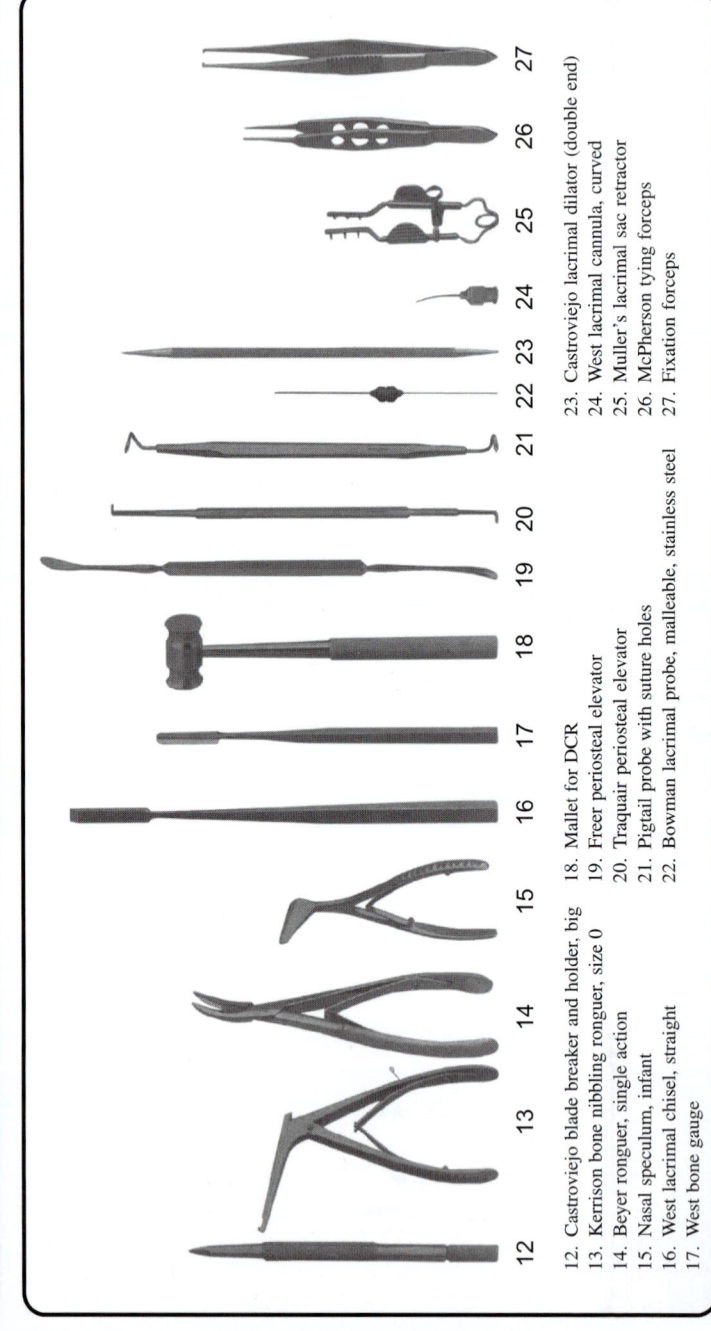

12. Castroviejo blade breaker and holder, big
13. Kerrison bone nibbling ronguer, size 0
14. Beyer ronguer, single action
15. Nasal speculum, infant
16. West lacrimal chisel, straight
17. West bone gauge
18. Mallet for DCR
19. Freer periosteal elevator
20. Traquair periosteal elevator
21. Pigtail probe with suture holes
22. Bowman lacrimal probe, malleable, stainless steel
23. Castroviejo lacrimal dilator (double end)
24. West lacrimal cannula, curved
25. Muller's lacrimal sac retractor
26. McPherson tying forceps
27. Fixation forceps

OTHERS

Strabismus Surgery Set

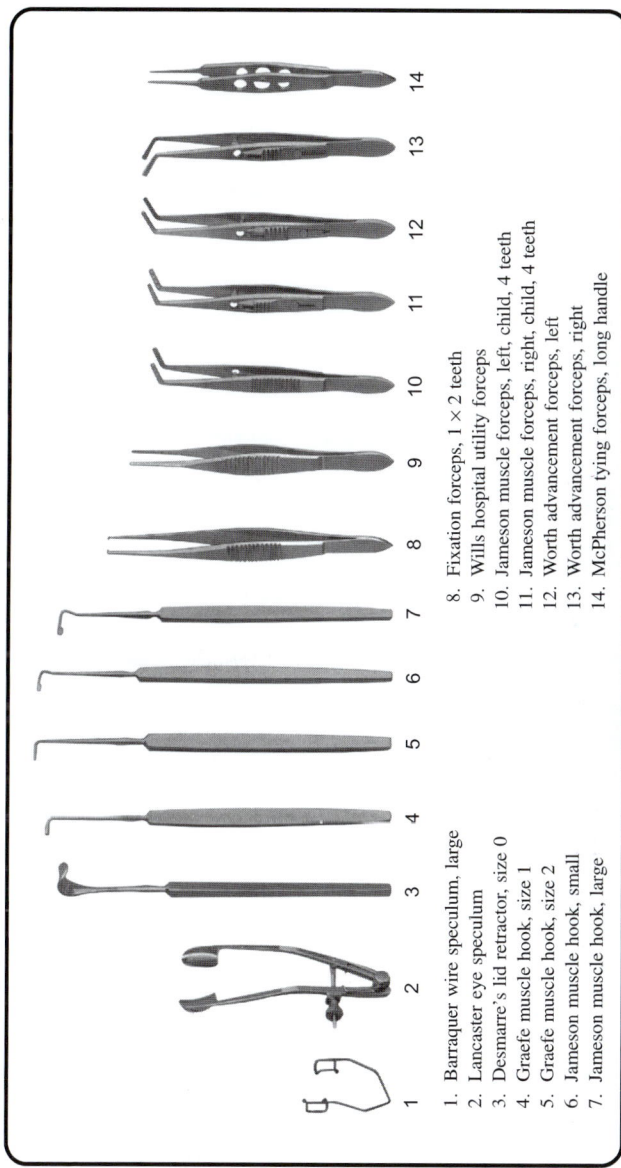

1. Barraquer wire speculum, large
2. Lancaster eye speculum
3. Desmarre's lid retractor, size 0
4. Graefe muscle hook, size 1
5. Graefe muscle hook, size 2
6. Jameson muscle hook, small
7. Jameson muscle hook, large
8. Fixation forceps, 1 × 2 teeth
9. Wills hospital utility forceps
10. Jameson muscle forceps, left, child, 4 teeth
11. Jameson muscle forceps, right, child, 4 teeth
12. Worth advancement forceps, left
13. Worth advancement forceps, right
14. McPherson tying forceps, long handle

Strabismus Surgery Set (contd.)

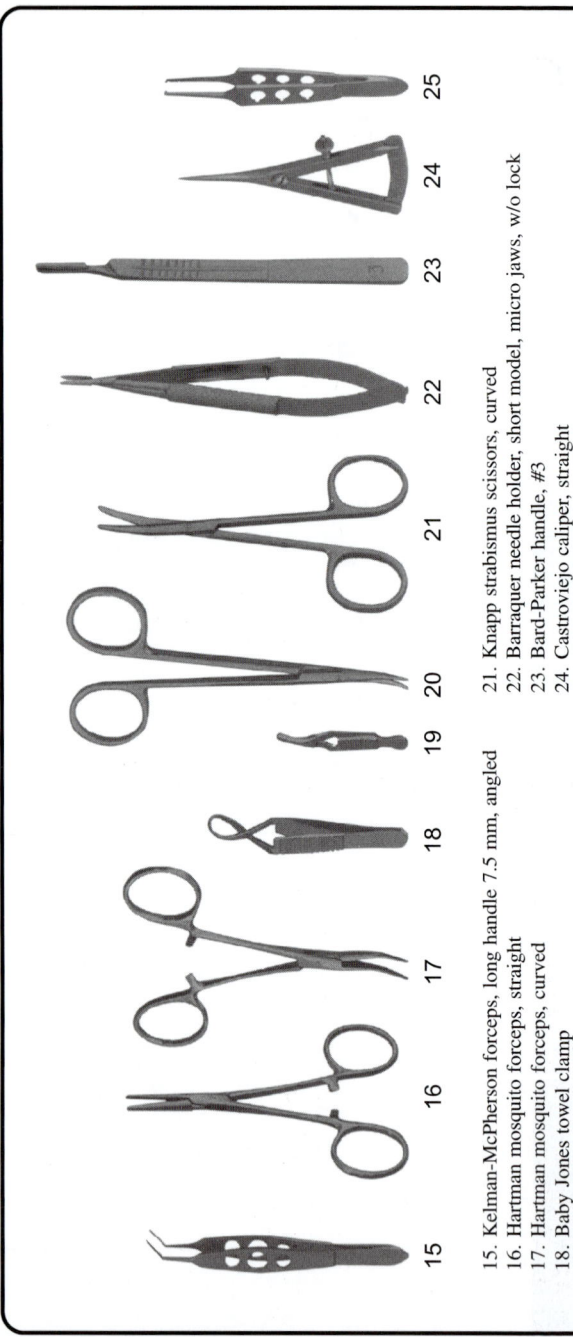

15. Kelman-McPherson forceps, long handle 7.5 mm, angled
16. Hartman mosquito forceps, straight
17. Hartman mosquito forceps, curved
18. Baby Jones towel clamp
19. Serrefine small, straight
20. Stevens tenotomy scissors, curved
21. Knapp strabismus scissors, curved
22. Barraquer needle holder, short model, micro jaws, w/o lock
23. Bard-Parker handle, #3
24. Castroviejo caliper, straight
25. Bishop Harmon forceps

Enucleation Set

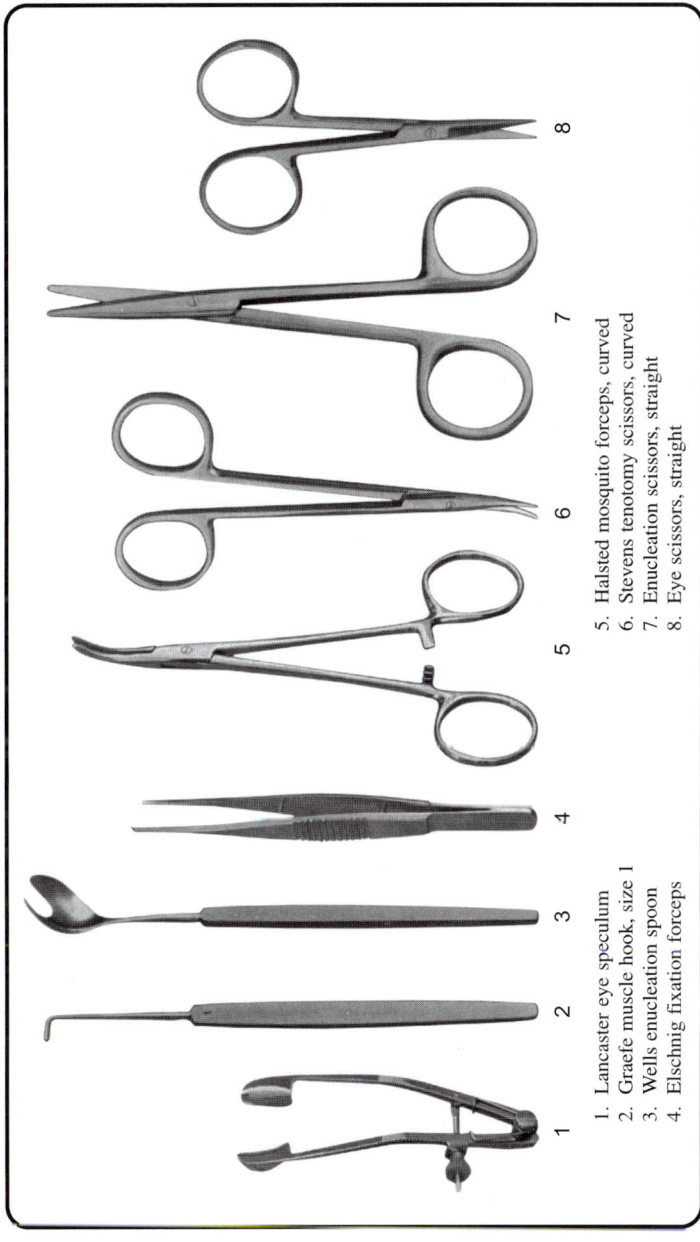

1. Lancaster eye speculum
2. Graefe muscle hook, size 1
3. Wells enucleation spoon
4. Elschnig fixation forceps
5. Halsted mosquito forceps, curved
6. Stevens tenotomy scissors, curved
7. Enucleation scissors, straight
8. Eye scissors, straight

INDEX